Gut Health for Women

6 Tips to Heal Your Gut, Optimize Digestion, Reduce Stress, and Balance Your Hormones Naturally

Aurora Bloom

Table of Contents

Introduction

If there's one thing to know about the human body: it's this: the human body has a ringmaster. This ringmaster controls your digestion, your immunity, your brain, your weight, your health and even your happiness. This ringmaster is your gut. –Nancy Mure

Lying awake at 1 a.m., unable to fall asleep quickly for another agonizing night, I turned on my side and stared at the wall. I thought of how most of my family and friends were probably sleeping soundly, and it filled me with sleep envy. Why do they get to sleep while I stay awake yet again? What's wrong with me? I felt confused. How could others fall asleep so easily while I spent hours counting sheep and listening to sleep apps through headphones? I felt despair as all the thoughts and stressors from the day ran through my head.

As I stared at the ceiling or the wall night after night, I knew something had to change. But what? If I couldn't pinpoint the problem, how could I fix anything? I started thinking about how sleep wasn't my only problem. I was stressed, irritable, and anxious. I felt like a hormonal teen all over again, but I was now in my thirties. I constantly thought to myself, I'm just a busy person and I need to adjust to this hectic life. I'll get there eventually. But my body didn't feel the same way. I was traveling a ton, eating on random schedules, partying and drinking a bit too much with friends, and not exercising as much as I needed to. No wonder my brain was reacting the way it was by not allowing me to settle down each night. Every evening I felt on edge and uneasy as bedtime approached. This feeling didn't help my sleeping habits at all. I started reacting with more anxiety each night as I lay in bed with my overactive brain. How long would it take to fall asleep tonight? Three hours… Four? Once I finally fell asleep, how long would I stay asleep? *Probably not long,* I told myself, which stressed me even more. This made me frustrated and unable to settle my thoughts. My brain was on overdrive each night, but I didn't know what to do to end this cycle. I spoke with others about my sleep issues sometimes, but it's difficult to talk about this when you feel like you're the only one experiencing it.

Now, it would be one thing if sleep was the only issue that I was trying to manage, but unfortunately, this was not the case. My body was also run-down, my brain seemed scattered, and I was constantly feeling overwhelmed and stressed. I tried to hide these feelings around other people and looked for quick fixes everywhere with fad diets and expensive supplements that I thought would take care of my problems. I was able to somewhat cope on the outside, but inside I worried that these feelings would never end, and I would never feel whole.

Finally, I reached my breaking point.

I was a few hours into a flight on an airplane when my first panic attack hit me. It was one of the worst experiences of my life because I truly didn't know what was happening or what had caused this feeling. My chest tightened, fingers clenching the seat, I was unable to catch my breath. I felt like I would vomit, and I was overheating while my thoughts raced. People were on the plane all around me, but I felt alone and didn't know what to do to feel steady and in control again. As I sweated profusely through my clothes, my thoughts quickly turned to ideas of death, and I panicked even more. I couldn't help it. When faced with this circumstance, I think many would feel the same way. I felt utterly disconnected from the world and just tried to breathe as I maintained eye contact with the seat in front of me.

At the moment, this experience felt like it would never end, but it finally passed, and I was able to calm down for the remainder of the flight. I did not leave my anxiety on the plane, however. Everything started getting worse at this point. Each day, I felt non-stop anxiousness and didn't know how to calm down. I found myself drinking more alcohol than I'd like to admit, but this only exacerbated the problem. Once I sobered up again, my mind and body felt terrible, and anxiety set in again. Truthfully, I didn't want to leave the house. I had suffered many other panic attacks during this time, and I was afraid that at any moment I would be hit again with another one. I didn't know where or when one would strike, and I was in a constant state of dread pondering the feelings I had with the first one. Even though I shared some of these feelings with others, I couldn't help feeling like I was becoming an inconvenience or a burden.

Something needed to change. When I started researching panic attacks more, I was able to put together more pieces of my anxiety puzzle. I was not just facing panic attacks, rather, the attacks were a result of the built-up stress and unhealthy habits my body had come to know. I knew I was not taking care of myself as I should but, when I started examining my lifestyle, all signs pointed to the sources and triggers for these attacks. Due to my eating and drinking habits, I felt slow and sluggish all the time. I had gained 15 pounds, which I could not shed regardless of how I ate or exercised. My sleep cycles were still a disaster, my muscles were sore and inflamed most days, and my belly felt puffy and bloated. This didn't help with my stress levels, but again, I wondered what I could do since I felt like I had to keep pushing myself with my busy lifestyle.

Eventually, I started seeing a doctor specializing in root cause treatments. I wanted to discover more about my ailments and get to the source of my anxiety. In the process, I found out that my immune system was working overtime to attack my thyroid and that, if I didn't change my habits, I would develop an autoimmune disease within the next several years. This news changed my life, and I knew I wouldn't be the same again.

I learned that I would need to cut gluten from my diet and change most of my nutritional habits. Needless to say, I was not super enthusiastic about the work I would have to do for this, but I also knew where I was headed if I didn't make some serious changes. So, what was the first thing I did? More research. I now have a desire to learn more about my health and new nutritional habits so that I could try to change my body both inside and out. What I discovered in doing this research is that the foods I needed to put into my body would not just help me physically, but mentally as well. So much of the way we think, behave, and function is a result of what we choose to eat every single day. Researching health became my passion and I wanted to know everything about how I could take control of my own. For hours, I would dive into articles, books, and podcasts, and a new world of discovery opened for me. This research, to some degree, already made me feel less anxious because I was taking small steps toward building a better relationship with food. Then, my world started to make sense as I learned about the gut-brain connection.

I completed a gut health course with a certified nutritionist and my passion for this subject continued. I then implemented the gut health theory into practice by making changes to the way I eat and live. To my surprise, I noticed significant improvements in my anxiety levels, fatigue, sleep, and just my overall well-being. Once my thoughts and practices around food changed, I felt rewarded in almost every area of my life.

I'd like to say this all happened overnight, but this was not the case. While I was surprised at the way I felt soon after changing my diet, this adventure was not without its setbacks. But, armed with a passion for learning about gut health and a desire to change the way I lived so that my stress would decrease and my body would feel better, I took steps to make changes over time.

For me, and for many people, this process is a journey. It takes motivation, consistency, and asking the right questions to stay on top of gut health.

Once I learned more about this topic, I became especially interested in focusing on women's struggles - with dieting, digestive issues, challenges with eating as a social aspect, and cultural standards that give us contradictory messages about weight loss and health. I now strive to put into words just how vital gut health is in our lives. This became a topic that I wanted to share with others and readers as they navigate through their own health journey. My goal is to present a straightforward, practical guidebook to rethinking the foods we eat, managing and reducing stress, and developing habits that benefit the body for improved gut health and general well-being. Like I said, there are many confusing and contradictory messages surrounding health and nutrition; with for-profit companies that exist to exploit diet culture, it becomes stressful and overwhelming trying to navigate this road. So, I want to share a simplified yet thorough guide to gut health that women can refer to as they adapt strategies and become the best, most vibrant versions of themselves.

Why This Matters

Now that I've had a chance to present my personal journey with gut health, you may feel that this information relates to some symptoms and struggles that you're currently facing. Please know that you're not alone! Whether you're dealing with all of these symptoms or just a few, we are going to work through them together in this book. Practicing good gut health is an ongoing part of my life, but it is rewarding and game changing. If you don't know where to start, this book is for you. If you're starting to learn about it but feel overwhelmed and need some encouragement, this book is still for you. If you're a pro and feel like you just need some practical reminders and assistance in continuing your personal journey, this book can still offer you guidance and helpful suggestions. I want to meet you at your current level and, with your personal goals in mind, help you achieve the health and mindset you wish for.

Regardless of where you are in your journey, please understand that what you put into your practice of gut health is what you will gain from it. Practicing the strategies outlined in this book will only be beneficial if you are taking specific steps to improve your lifestyle. Make this journey your own so that you get the most from it and allow me to be your "hype-woman" along the path to an improved lifestyle. I found that once I had a sense of how to improve my gut health, the pieces of other areas of my life started falling into place as well. This is my hope for readers. I want you to feel vibrant, healthy, and alive again. I want you to have the information and understanding so that you can make gut health a priority in your life. I also want you to have the best sleep, skin, digestion, and mental health that you've ever experienced. I come to you with openness and honesty about how I continue on my path to improved gut health, and I'd like you to apply the information provided so that you're able to have an engaging experience for yourself. I'm with you, supporting you every step of the way. So, let's get started on your journey with love, kindness, and understanding.

Medical Disclaimer

While the information in this book has been researched, it is not intended to replace the professional advice of a medical physician. If you have any concerns with your own health or well-being regarding gut health, it is always best to consult professionals in the area of healthcare so they can prescribe the most effective and personalized diagnosis and treatment.

Chapter 1:

Gut Health and You

Consider your daily routine for a moment. Most people are busy and work to keep up with tasks they need to accomplish but take some time now to think about the jobs you take on every day. If you'd like, take a moment to make a list of these, as this may help put into perspective exactly how many hats you wear daily. For example, are you employed and do you have various roles with your company? Are you a caretaker for someone (even pets)? Are you in charge of managing a home and setting appointments for yourself and others? These are simply a few ideas to get you started in considering how much you are responsible for each day. If you think about and list how many jobs you may take on within a day, week, month, or year, this will probably confirm that you are a busy person working to keep up with your roles and assignments.

While making this list can seem overwhelming, it is meant to pinpoint just how important self-care and nutrition are so that you can keep up with the many tasks you complete. You may know your body well enough to understand that you cannot take on certain tasks while you're hungry. Your body needs some nourishment to function properly. But, for many, we're so busy that we grab the closest snack or fastest meal so we can keep going through our day. Often, we're simply looking for a way to push through the next hour or two without stopping to consider how the foods we consume will make us feel in the long term.

This is the mindset that we will start to rethink as we focus on gut health. There are small steps that individuals can take immediately to change their diets for the better. This simply requires knowledge and practice. Once you know about gut health and why it's so important for basic functions of the body, you'll be able to apply this information to your everyday lives.

The Gut Overview

So, let's begin with an explanation of what gut health is and why it's so vital to our well-being. The idea of "gut health" covers all areas related to the digestive system, from the esophagus to the bowel. These are the parts responsible for breaking down our food and creating energy for our bodies so we can function effectively. Each area of the gut has a specific and important job to complete as colonies of microorganisms help digest the foods we put into our bodies (Mudge, 2022). So, with this information in mind, gut health should be easy, right? If we simply eat the foods, we've been told to eat from any food pyramid we've viewed in the past, we're good, right? Well, while gut health does center on including a variety of foods in the diet, there is much more to it than just focusing on food groups.

True gut health places a focus on the brain and body working in conjunction with each other. If the right foods are not consumed, functions break down and leave us feeling sluggish and mentally drained. When nourishing foods are eaten, we can achieve peak performance and mental clarity. It sounds great, doesn't it? So why isn't everyone doing this? Why aren't people shouting from the rooftops that we need to eat the right foods that will benefit our gut health the most? Well, for the same reasons that diets tend to fade and people return to old habits. Maintaining motivation is challenging for most people, especially when life ramps up and we need quick meals to get us through the day. That's why putting a personalized plan in place for your gut health will be crucial as you consider ways to feel your best. But we'll get there. First, we need to examine more about the importance of gut health and its benefits. So, take note of the following to gain some drive and motivation on your journey.

A body that prioritizes gut health can see and feel improvements in (Dehbi, 2019):

- digestion.

- maintaining a healthy weight.

- sleep.

- stress reduction.

- increased energy levels.

- clearer skin.

- gastrointestinal issues.

- happiness (Yes, that's right! This is an important one that we'll get to!).

- balanced hormone levels.

The Gut Microbiome

If you research any information about gut health, you will quickly discover a word that is at the core (literally) of an individual's gut, the microbiome. Simply put, this term refers to "the community of microorganisms (such as fungi, bacteria, and viruses) that exist in a particular environment" (Segre,

2022). These are the microorganisms that assist in absorbing nutrients in the body, digesting fibers and foods for energy, and controlling the immune system as well as brain health. Needless to say, these are important instruments for functioning well, but how many times a day do you even consider the importance of your digestive tract? I'd venture to say that you probably don't give it much thought until something feels wrong and you have a digestive problem. I certainly didn't think much about digestive health until I started learning more about its significance. If you've ever had an upset stomach, nausea, constipation, or diarrhea, and, let's face it, most of us have, you understand the feelings that can be associated with these issues. At the moment, these symptoms feel like they will never improve or disappear. Well, guess what? Sometimes they won't until we decide to take action on our gut health. We can often mask symptoms with chewables, chalky drinks, and medications, but these are temporary solutions to a much bigger and ongoing problem. You may have heard this before and laughed it off, but our gut really is like a second brain within our bodies.

Unlike the big brain in your skull, the enteric nervous system (ENS) can't organize your finances or write a love note. "Its main role is controlling digestion, from swallowing to the release of enzymes that break down food to the control of blood flow that helps with nutrient absorption to elimination," explains Jay Pasricha, M.D., director of the Johns Hopkins Center for Neurogastroenterology, whose research on the enteric nervous system has garnered international attention. (*The Brain-Gut Connection*, 2019).

The digestive tract acts as the source of many problems when it's not cared for, from diarrhea to depression. Knowing this can also help us understand how gut health is directly linked to brain health. Brain chemicals like serotonin and dopamine, the ones that control so much of our mood and happiness, are influenced by how our gut bacteria are absorbing the right foods (Embracing Nutrition, 2019). It's no wonder then that poor gut health can be linked to feelings of depression and anxiety. Sufferers of Irritable Bowel Syndrome (IBS) and other digestive illnesses often report higher levels of anxiety and depression.

For women, issues with digestion seem to be even more problematic. Let's face it, women carry a ton of responsibilities in this world. You probably know women (or are one) who have continued caring for family members even while they, themselves, are sick or exhausted. While having the martyr mentality is not necessarily a healthy mindset, it is ingrained in our culture to be a "warrior woman." When it comes to digestive health for women, the gut unfortunately often takes a backseat to other more pressing matters. According to Dr. Vora, "In particular with women's gut health, I think a lot of women have resigned themselves to having chronic gut dysfunction, thinking it's inevitable or related to something seemingly out of their control, such as their menstrual cycle or their stress levels" (Well + Good Editors, 2019). The result of this for many women is to simply normalize not feeling healthy when it comes to digestion. Feeling unhealthy should never be normalized. Because of these ideas, many people assume they must live with discomfort, pain, illness, sleep deprivation, and more.

Searching for Solutions

To combat the misnomers surrounding gut health, people need to be more open about discussing this topic. After all, digestion is important in so many areas of life. When we feel slowed down or sick from the foods we eat, it makes sense that we should take control of the situation. But what about times when we feel okay or we're simply too busy to change our eating habits and would rather spend time on other aspects of our lives? This is understandable, after all, since learning to eat the right foods can take some time and adjustments. For example, if you've always eaten certain sugars, starches, or proteins, it may take more motivation to rethink the current foods you think you love. This becomes especially challenging when you feel like you'll miss the foods you won't eat anymore. Instead of feeling like you're limiting yourself by cutting out certain foods—think of this as a way to test how you feel and how your body reacts to the deliciously healthy foods you will soon eat.

Knowing which foods are the "right foods" for this digestive journey makes a difference in the way a person can plan and think about gut health. If you're reading this, you've probably experienced a need to consider your digestive health, whether it be due to something serious like an illness or something seemingly simplistic like an occasional upset stomach. Regardless of what your body is feeling at this time, it's important to know the symptoms and triggers of your digestive issues. Just as you would gauge and monitor your results after being prescribed a new medication by your doctor, start monitoring the foods you know may be the root cause of problems for you. Take some time, even weeks or months, to make a list of these because, most likely, there is a tasty replacement that will satisfy your craving for the former food. Once you begin eating the right gut-healthy nutrients, your body will start to recalibrate to adjust to this new way, and you may find the cravings are no longer there.

I'll be honest, this road may be tough. Learning about gut health may challenge you to rethink your old ways. For me, my motivation was my desire to feel physically better so that my body wouldn't be triggered and return to panic mode. My long-term health was and still is very important to me, so I now prioritize this. Because people need to find better ways of ensuring that poor gut health doesn't take control of their bodies and moods, they need to understand the benefits of having and maintaining a healthy gut.

Gut Health and Hormones

Especially for women, ensuring that our gut health is at its peak performance is an excellent way to balance hormones naturally. When we don't eat foods that will encourage proper gut health, our gut can have a large influence on stress levels and decision-making. To regulate neurotransmitters and the messages that are sent between the brain and the body, we need to ensure that we are taking care of our gut bacteria so that it works in our favor. When these bacteria are fed starchy carbs, sugars, and certain fats, they go to work on our insides in all the wrong ways. If you've ever felt sad or angry once you've come down from a sugar high, for example, you can start to gain an understanding and appreciation for just how in control the gut is over our mood and feelings.

While the advice and suggestions offered in this book could benefit anyone, because my experience specifically centers on my connection as a woman who dealt with digestive issues for years, I will share more of my expertise on women's health. Since gut health plays a large role in women's hormone levels, it's important to note here that much of my research is geared toward assisting a woman on her journey to better health. To do this, it's necessary to understand how the gut directly impacts a woman's body. Several serious health issues that are specific to females can arise as a result of poor gut health.

When gut health isn't optimal, hormones become imbalanced. For example, there is new research showing that the microbiome plays a big role in estrogen regulation. These studies indicate that poor gut health increases the risk of estrogen-related diseases such as Polycystic Ovary Syndrome (PCOS), endometriosis, and even breast cancer (Scott, n.d.).

Because estrogen levels assist with cognitive, bone, and cardiovascular health, it's important to consider how improved hormone levels may allow a person to feel more energized, happy, and in control of their surroundings. While supplements can help with hormone replacement and regulation, maintaining a healthy diet is one of the most important ways to ensure that a person's body will be balanced.

When healthy foods are absorbed in the gut and used to satisfy and energize an individual, it has a positive impact on the organs of the human body as well (just another plus to practicing good gut health!). When you eat, the stomach and intestines help absorb the food into the bloodstream, which leads to many areas of the body where these nutrients can work their magic. The liver is one of these important places where, with the right foods, this organ can remove harmful disease-causing toxins from the body (Francis, 2021). When this happens successfully, the gut and liver are working together to be as efficient with those food nutrients as possible. When this doesn't take place, however, a person becomes more susceptible to illness and disease after some time. Eating organic whole foods will help with the proper absorption of these nutrients and balance that liver-gut connection. In a future chapter, we'll explore more of the healthy foods that can recharge and rebalance a diet.

At this stage, you may be feeling inundated with a myriad of information about gut health. Well, the reality is that this topic is one of the most important medical health issues and it is not discussed enough. With your new knowledge about what it encompasses and why it's so important, let's take our journey to the next level. Discovering the signs, causes, and effects of poor digestion can help you pinpoint the areas of your diet that may need the most attention. You'll learn information about how you can recognize any poor habits you may currently have so that you can change them and be on your way to better health. This change does not need to take place today (although it absolutely can), but by learning the causes and effects of poor gut health, you'll have the power to start making decisions about and taking control of your body. So, let's get started!

Chapter 2:

Signs, Causes, and Effects of

Poor Gut Health

All disease begins in the gut. –Hippocrates

It's time to discuss some of the harsh truths associated with the gut. Picture this scenario:

You're rushing to work because you've had a hectic morning stuck in traffic. You've quickly eaten a processed breakfast bar in the car on your way, and now you're pulling into the parking lot while quickly guzzling the last sips of the coffee you brought from home. You realize you're about to be late for a meeting, so you rush inside and head to the conference room. For a second, all seems calm and you've made it on time, so you grab a seat and prepare. Ten minutes into the meeting, you notice it. There's a bloated, uncomfortable feeling in your stomach that's building up. You move around nonchalantly in your seat for a moment, hoping no one will hear your stomach gurgle. A few more minutes pass, and by now you're just hoping that the meeting will be shorter than expected, but you have no idea how long it will be until you can get to the bathroom—more bloating. More discomfort. By now, you're starting to sweat and your heart is racing faster, partly because you feel uncomfortable and partly because you're nervous that your body is going to start making some unplanned sounds. You hope no one around you notices the beads of sweat on your forehead. Finally, you can't take it anymore. You stand up

"

in front of everyone and shuffle out of the room quickly so you can make it to the bathroom in time. Crisis averted, but embarrassment avoided? Not so much.

Before we get to the positive aspects of gut health, it's necessary to examine some of the catalysts that place so many people in stressful positions to make decisions about getting healthier with their gut. You may feel like you understand your body well enough to make informed decisions about what is causing you to feel sick or simply not as strong as you could feel, but can you truly pinpoint what measures to take before a digestive situation gets out of control? It's here that we need to learn what signs to look for so that we can understand the effect that our choices have on our bodies every day. So, let's next take a look at some of the problems so that, with time and change, we can see the solutions on the horizon.

What Is "Poor Gut Health?"

No one tries to have certain digestive issues on purpose, right? For various reasons, many people end up in a place where they know what they should eat and drink or what exercises and self-care they should practice, but don't apply this regularly (or sometimes ever). We get busy and we indulge from time to time, rarely considering the consequences, because we just want to live. The strange aspect of this tends to be that it's our poor habits and practices that hold us back from our ability to live. Imagine, for example, not exercising for months or even years and then expecting your body to be able to run a 26-mile marathon. Our bodies would hate us for doing that to them, so why do we expect them to feel fine after majorly processed foods or insane amounts of sugar? Part of the answer here is that most of us are conditioned to live in a culture where these substances are all around us. We're brought up to believe that because certain foods are approved to be sold at stores and consumed by the public, we don't need to think twice about what we're putting into our bodies. Because products sell and companies make a profit, this will most likely, and unfortunately, be a controlling part of our world for an indefinite amount of time.

So, what can be done about this? Well, there are ways to rebel against these traditional methods of thinking about our health and make progress as an individual, but we need to look at the basics of poor gut health first. What is it and what is holding us back from feeling better?

Causes of Poor Gut Health

Simply put, when bad bacteria in our gut is allowed to thrive, we won't feel well. The microbes that are in the intestinal tract help us obtain energy from foods, eliminate toxins, fight viruses, and produce serotonin for a mood boost (*Signs of Poor Gut Health*, n.d.). If you've suffered from poor gut health and started researching your symptoms, you've probably encountered talk of gluten, a protein found in wheat, rye, and barley, which many people track as a source of a problem for gut health (McDonald, 2020). While this is not the only substance to blame, it can cause inflammation and poor digestion. Of course, seeing a doctor is always best when working to pinpoint a problem with gut health, but you may also want to start tracking how you feel after you eat certain foods, especially foods that contain gluten, to see if there is any correlation here.

As mentioned in the discussion about identifying obstacles and setbacks to gut health, processed foods are another common problem leading to poor gut health. These foods very often cause inflammation in the gut, leading to bloating or sick feelings after they are consumed. For many people, if the problem is minor, they may simply try to deal with this feeling after they eat, not realizing that the feeling may be eliminated completely by avoiding certain foods.

High-stress levels are also, naturally, not good for gut health. Everyone, to some degree, will encounter stress throughout their life, but understanding methods to help calm nerves, adjust to change, and care for oneself can make a major difference in the way our gut reacts to stress. Because the brain and gut are so closely linked, for many, life interruptions can cause an upset stomach or other symptoms. Knowing how to notice feelings of stress is useful for understanding the tools that one can use to relieve stress and feel both physically and mentally capable and confident.

Because poor gut health can have such a large impact on the body, it's important to also understand some of the lesser-known causes of digestive issues. These include surprising sources that, for some, could require a simple change to a person's eating habits. For example, neglecting a diverse range of foods, lacking prebiotics or probiotics, or overindulging in alcohol or cigarettes can all lead to poor gut health (Coyle, 2017). To observe and make changes in this area, start by getting in tune with the factors that trigger you when feeling poorly. Feeling 'unhealthy' can mean feeling sick on a physical level or simply feeling worn out, tired, angry, or any other emotion that may hold a person back from accomplishing tasks well. Often, humans like to mask real problems with food, alcohol, or other drugs, but these typically provide only temporary relief from real issues. To reach the core of the problem, one may need to experiment with eliminating certain foods and incorporating subtle healthy additions to a diet and lifestyle that will make effective changes.

Signs and Symptoms

The signs that will come with poor gut health could take many forms, such as hormonal imbalances, fatigue, stomach discomfort, weight changes, allergies, autoimmune deficiencies, migraines, acne, and other life-altering conditions (Patino, 2020). Again, if you notice any negative signs or changes in your symptoms, seek medical advice to start understanding why certain issues may be occurring. For me, this journey of researching and learning more from my doctors made a positive difference in my ability to receive help and make the changes I needed to make. If you feel that you are currently suffering from one or more of the symptoms described, reach out to your physician for more information.

Ultimately, when we're lacking good bacteria in our gut, this issue can cause depression, sluggishness, anxiety, irritable bowel syndrome, sleep issues, and even skin allergies. This is not to say that these issues will always be the result of depriving the gut of good foods, but these are some of the most common results that need attention and focus. Experiencing several of these symptoms at once can also occur, as one symptom may lead to another over time. Bloating, diarrhea, and "leaky gut" can result from poor gut health. Leaky gut syndrome occurs when the gut lining has been injured and can lead to intestinal permeability over time if left untreated. Stress, poor diet, or injuries can wear down the intestinal lining, causing permeability (*Leaky Gut Syndrome*, 2022).

Certain symptoms associated with leaky gut can also lead to more chronic problems, like a constant lack of sleep, loss of appetite, and a sense of urgency before using the bathroom. These life interruptions are serious when they impact the amount of time we spend with loved ones and when these symptoms interfere with our careers. Taking control of these symptoms to have the ability to improve your life is needed so that long-term conditions don't develop. If you are having any abnormal bowel movements, skin irritations, allergies, fatigue, or mood issues, consider how your diet may be a triggering factor for these conditions.

For women specifically, hormonal changes or imbalances can impact the timing of a menstrual cycle, so simple blood and urine tests can indicate if there is an issue impacting gut health in conjunction with this. Weight gain, low sex drive, thinning hair, increased thirst or hunger, and excessive sweating often go hand-in-hand with hormonal changes (*Do You Have a Hormonal Imbalance?*, 2022). Researching the symptoms you experience and finding sources that you feel comfortable using, such as at-home testing or a visit to a doctor or naturopath, can help you understand more about your personal situation.

Long-Term Impact

For many people, visiting a doctor and discussing "private matters" when it comes to digestion may be challenging. We want to move on with our day instead of putting time into noticing the symptoms that we may be suffering from. It's important to discuss such issues with a physician before the symptoms become a serious problem, but if you are already experiencing a condition, understand that it's not too late to take steps toward action and do something to change your health. This is important for many reasons, but one of the main ones is to understand the possible long-term impacts of poor gut health. Depression, Parkinson's and Alzheimer's disease, Multiple Sclerosis, and strokes can be long-term results of ignoring important health needs (Gardiner, 2021). Neuroinflammation, or an inflammatory response in the brain or spinal cord caused by aging, poor health, and cell decay, can occur when gut health issues are left untreated (DiSabato et al., 2016). To combat this, it's important to know the right items that will help your body stay as healthy as possible for as long as possible. In the next section, we'll get into the nitty-gritty of how to eliminate foods that don't serve you well and how to read food labels so we can avoid inflammatory ingredients.

Chapter 3:

Tip#1—Cut It Out

Balance in the body is the foundation for balance in life. –B.K.S. Iyengar

In this chapter, we'll start focusing on the foods that may be holding you back. If you consider yourself a fairly healthy eater, you may have already encountered some of the pieces of information presented here. Even if you make an effort to consciously choose and eliminate certain items from your diet, there is always something to learn when it comes to gut health. First, I'd like to remind you to please keep an open mind.

Try not to think of taking care of your gut as having to cut most of the things that you love from your diet. Instead, consider the foods that you currently eat and examine the ingredients to decide if they are right for you or if there are any alternatives or substitutions that you can implement on your journey to improved gut health.

Moving ahead, let's examine how to eliminate ingredients that cause inflammation or may be holding you back from feeling your best. My goal is to provide you with a wealth of information to guide you on a path to making better choices for your health.

Typically, the hardest thing about traditional 'dieting' is feeling a sense of deprivation, but with the knowledge you'll gain, you'll have a better understanding of the delicious variety of foods that can be incorporated into eating well. The first step in healing the gut is to stop eating the things that make you feel unhealthy and sick. So, here we go with Tip #1: Cut It Out.

This section will provide a straightforward guide to what can be done today to begin a healthier lifestyle.

The Truth About Diets

You're in a large room with 100 people for one hour. Your task is to mingle around the room, talking to as many different people as possible to get a better sense of what their personalities are like. You begin by interacting with the first person, and they start saying how much they hate what you're wearing today. You decide to move on to the next person. You introduce yourself to them and they talk about the sunny, delightful weather that they see through the window. The third person you walk up to compliments you on your outfit and starts asking you questions to get to know you better, seemingly interested in what you will say. You continue wandering around the room for an hour, meeting some individuals who are polite and some who you would never want to encounter again. Then, the experiment is over. You're asked to reflect on the different interactions you just had with people and how they made you feel. You conclude that you felt better and happier when talking to positive individuals, and you felt anxious and terrible when talking with those who were negative and unkind.

Now, consider this room as a metaphor for your stomach. The foods you put into it will interact with each other and with the environment that they're placed in. Some will get along, some will not. Some will make you feel energized and some will make you want to shut down. Think of your digestive tract as a place where many foods and nutrients have to coincide. Sometimes, the reaction to your body and mind will be great, but not always. Typically, when we understand more about what impacts our system, we can learn from this and make better choices in the future. Think about people in your life that you may have encountered who were rude or mean to you in the past. Do you feel like you want to continue spending time with these people, and do you seek out moments where you can meet up? Reactions to foods can be similar. If you've ever experienced a food allergy or became sick from eating or drinking a certain item, you may now have negative feelings about that thing when you think about it. For many, becoming violently ill from a food or liquid is often all it takes to eliminate this food or beverage from their diet. Gut health is tricky, though, and many times, it's hard to pinpoint the culprit because it's difficult to justify eliminating something that only makes us mildly ill.

I believe that it's important to know and understand what kinds of ingredients cause inflammation and irritation to the gut. These could be the foods that are subtly harmful, but over time can lead to more serious issues. Readers, please know that I do not believe in traditional 'diets,' hence the quotation marks when I write about them. I think they feel like quick fixes that are not sustainable, whereas, what I'd like to encourage more is a lifestyle alteration. Those people crammed into that room together could never get along perfectly at all times, so why do we try to force the unhealthy items into the same room as the healthy ones and expect to feel fine afterward?

This is not to say that the complete elimination of the less healthy items is the perfect answer either. Adding more of the healthy options, though, will eventually overpower some of the negativity in the digestive tract, just as more positive, healthy attitudes in a room full of people may outweigh the few negative, toxic personalities. If it helps, start thinking of your stomach this way. There are competing foods that you will put in, but the more you focus on adding good foods to your menu each day, the more your body will adapt to accepting and absorbing the positive nutrients as it starts digesting in a healthier way.

The Food Journey

When I started focusing on eliminating the bad and adding the good to my personal food journey, I noticed something. I realized that I was able to tune into my body more so that I could listen to and learn from it. I tracked the items that made me feel bad or that physically caused me to react in a certain way, such as bloating or fatigue. Noting these reactions gave me a sense of power. I was able to choose and accept any consequences of that choice. I balanced the effect of the food with how badly I wanted to eat it.

Sometimes this wasn't easy, and I didn't always make the healthiest choices, but I continued to try. After I understood the effect the food would have on my body, I was able to work harder on the elimination process. I cut out gluten and dairy products, and as a result, I started feeling different, better, and healthier.

For your personal journey, make decisions for yourself that will make the most sense in your day-to-day life. If a food doesn't make you feel well after eating it, weigh the pros and cons of eating it again. I believe in allowing yourself to enjoy meals as long as conscious decision-making is a part of this process. As with anything, moderation and management may be the keys. Obviously, if a certain food is harming you, complete elimination of it may be the only way to feel good. I will occasionally take a digestive enzyme before the rare occasions when I eat gluten or dairy so that my body is much better equipped to manage these items. Make the best decisions for yourself and remember that eating the right ingredients can, in its own way, be a form of self-care for treating bloating, fatigue, nausea, or even facial breakouts.

Some of the foods to consider eliminating may be the ones that irritate the bowels because they are highly processed. Again, many people in society are trained to think that it's perfectly fine to frequently eat things like these, even though the truth is that they have an enormous impact on the gut. Many of these same people often wonder why they're overweight, feeling a lack of motivation for everyday tasks, or coping with a major illness. Many of these processed foods will encourage the growth of bad bacteria in the gut and not give healthy bacteria a chance to thrive. Often, items that contain pesticides or herbicides, or some that are genetically modified, will also stimulate the growth of this harmful bacteria, so it's best to pay close attention to the individual food triggers that are causing harm and try to avoid them when possible (Giambò et al., 2021).

My goal is not to scare anyone with this research, but to encourage them to investigate and experiment with their own elimination diet because this can be the best learning tool. Fair warning that this kind of trial-and-error experimentation can take some time and can be challenging depending on individual needs, so again, incorporate this into your life in a way that makes the most sense for you. I will provide you with easy-to-follow, step-by-step ideas in this process. The first step is to learn to become more intuitive with your body. Start paying attention to what you eat and how it makes you feel. That's it. If you start doing this regularly, you will already be miles ahead of where most individuals are because you will have eliminated the mindless eating that so many people engage in daily.

The Elimination 'Diet'

The worst part of any diet is that feeling that you're missing out on something. This causes many to give up quickly and return to old habits. Our brains, many times, are no help with this either. We think we need something we are missing out on, and our minds go into panic mode. This kind of feeling can last for quite a while when a person diets, leading many to quit the diet and feel defeated later. Try keeping a food tracking journal to help you stay motivated and accountable on this journey. Simply making a list on your phone of what you eat and how you feel afterward can help you better understand which ingredients you may want to eliminate.

'Diet' is a strong word for what you can embark on when seeking improved gut health. Think of this instead as a discovery. You are the researcher, and you get to decide what will be best for you. This is the only way your mind is going to embrace any changes and turn these ideas into life-long progress. When you set yourself up for success, you are much more likely to continue, so begin with a positive attitude that does not involve depriving yourself. The goal is not starvation; instead, it is experimentation. "An elimination diet is a diagnostic and treatment tool to help discover any trigger foods that cause gastrointestinal symptoms as well as other symptoms such as headaches, rashes, joint pain, and brain fog" (Ruscio, 2021). This type of eating gives the body a recovery period so that it can reset. This process involves the temporary elimination (trial and error style) of food that you or your doctor suspect is triggering your symptoms and pausing your consumption of it to see how you feel. Needless to say, it's important to have some food triggers in mind before you begin the process of eliminating them so that you can track what may be causing problems. This method is not to identify allergies to foods, but rather to guide a person to more mindful eating once the trigger foods are reintroduced into the body. After two or three weeks, the idea is to slowly reintroduce the items that were eliminated back into your system so you can examine how these things make you feel when trying to digest them. While you're in this discovery phase, try to also focus on adding healthier foods to your day. Once the body starts adjusting to this, however, you may surprise yourself with the lack of cravings you notice for the processed items you once wanted. This is because your digestive tract is starting to reset itself. It's like a power button for your gut. When you reintroduce certain things that you feel may have triggered you before, you can decide how much and how often to consume them.

The Gluten and Dairy Dilemma

In life, you've probably known someone first-hand who is gluten or dairy intolerant. In fact, this issue has become so common that many food companies and restaurants address it by including gluten-free or dairy-free options for the public. There is a reason why we tend to hear so much about these two substances. For many, they are difficult to digest. Meals with gluten or dairy tend to interact with the gut in a not-so-pleasant way, causing bad bacteria to form. If you experiment with gluten and dairy during an elimination period, you may find that reintroducing these to the system has an impact on the gut. Many feel that these are two groups to be mindful of as they tend to cause irregularities in digestion. If you notice a problem as these are reintroduced, consider limiting or eliminating them from your diet and take note of any changes you notice.

Start getting in the habit of checking labels when you shop for groceries or ask about ingredients when eating at restaurants to educate yourself about foods that may include gluten or dairy. You may be surprised that it appears in so many menu items, but you may also be surprised at how many alternative options are starting to be offered as a result of a larger population inquiring about gluten and dairy.

Interestingly enough, over 65% of the world's population can't digest lactose, the sugar found in dairy products (Lindemann, 2016). In many cases, people who think they may be allergic to dairy are experiencing an inability to properly absorb lactose in their system. For these people, ingesting dairy can cause diarrhea, "leaky gut," or continued bloating, leading to much discomfort after consuming dairy products. If this sounds familiar and you suspect dairy to be a catalyst for the way you feel, try removing this from your diet to see what changes take place. At times, taking a digestive enzyme before you decide to consume cheese or other dairy products can be a good way to avoid an upset stomach. Eating raw or organic cheeses instead of processed ones can feel easier on the digestive system, so this may be a way to still enjoy cheese if that's something you crave.

Foods to Avoid

Since you're now starting to understand that some foods will upset the digestive tract and are best to avoid, you're probably on your way to personalizing a menu so that you can experiment with certain options for yourself. Besides gluten and dairy, there are some other major items to try to eliminate to notice if there's any impact on the way you feel.

Processed foods, including processed meats, often cause bad bacteria to continue to live in the system. "Advanced glycation end products (AGEs) are harmful compounds that are formed when protein or fat combine with sugar in the bloodstream" (Brown, 2019). Processed meats are a major source of these AGEs, and eliminating processed items in general, can be the best way to remove them from the body. Fast foods are especially notorious for containing processed meats, cheeses, and sugars, which are all substances that can cause gut problems and may be worth avoiding completely.

Sugars like cane syrup, table sugar (sucrose), high fructose corn syrup, and even artificial sweeteners like aspartame and sucralose can cause harm to the system. Sugar is often found in many everyday items we eat, so it's worth reading labels to start getting in the habit of noticing the quantity of sugar in foods. Eating sugar can lead to bigger problems like weight gain and other risky health conditions, including certain diseases (Spritzler, 2019). In addition to commonly known sweet foods, sugar is found in many alcoholic drinks. When this excess of sugar runs through the body and into the gut, humans get a temporary feeling of satisfaction and relief, only to soon feel a crash afterward. If you've ever become sleepy, irritable, or impatient after consuming things with sugar or alcoholic beverages, you now may understand why. Sugars give a "quick fix high," and then leave the body feeling slow, sluggish, angry, anxious, and deprived.

Let's get down to business on some of the more subtle inflammation-causing ingredients to avoid. Some lesser-known items can be harmful, but because they seem benign, they are often overlooked when discovering what foods to experiment with and what foods to avoid. Refined oils and refined carbs are two food groups that would seem okay for consumption when, in actuality, they can harm the system and help bad bacteria grow. Omega-rich foods used to be all the rage because they provide that "good oil" that is beneficial to digestion in the body. While this is true, these oils still need to be consumed in moderation, and refined oils like canola, sunflower, soybean, and corn can cause the system harm when they are included in meals too often (*Are Omega-6 Fatty Acids Linked to Heart Disease?*, 2021). The same is true for white bread, white pasta, cakes, and pastries, which quickly turn into sugar in our bodies.

Food Labels 101

Reading ingredient labels proves to be invaluable when it comes to understanding personalized nutrition. These labels provide key information and insight into how healthy or unhealthy a portion is for an individual. Many people obsess over the number of calories or the amount of fat in items while reading labels when, in reality, they should be focused on the list of ingredients. Ingredient names that you can recognize are where it's at! If you notice synthetic, processed items or unrecognizable substances on the label, this food is probably not healthy. If you see many naturally occurring items, whole foods, and minimal ingredients on the label instead, this food is most likely a healthier choice. Your body will naturally know how to digest these simpler foods and will not have to work overtime to absorb any nutrients you're consuming. A good rule of thumb is to remember that the fewer ingredients in the list, the better. If you don't know what the ingredient is, your body probably won't know how to digest it.

Get into the habit of checking for fiber and low sugar when looking at labels instead of focusing on calories. Pay attention to added artificial sugars, as these items have less nutritional value for your body and can wreak havoc on your gut. It's important to even be mindful of the amount of natural sugar in a product, as this can draw water into the large intestine and prevent foods from being absorbed properly (Hills, 2019). On ingredient labels, the majority of that food is going to appear as the first item, so if sugar is in the top ingredients, beware!

Another misnomer revolves around the words "all-natural." Natural foods are "foods that are free of synthetic or artificial ingredients or additives" (*Differences in Organic, Natural, and Health Foods*, 2021). While this can be a good thing, the term all-natural doesn't automatically make a food healthy. The same is true for foods advertised as "gluten-free." This phrase does not always mean healthier, and many times, gluten-free items will contain many harmful additives and preservatives. Knowing the food source, process, and ingredients can help in making more educated decisions.

The "Dirty Dozen"

I personally buy as much organic produce as possible because the foods that are grown organically tend to be better for our health. I realize that not every person has access to or the means to purchase organic items for their families and, while eating organic produce may not be a reality every day, I believe it should be considered when possible. Ultimately, when these are sprayed with pesticides and herbicides or are genetically modified, the fruits and vegetables that would normally be considered healthy can become harmful to our health and digestive system.

Below, I am including a list of the "dirty dozen," which is a guide to the produce you should make an effort to buy organically when you can (Environmental Working Group, 2019). Typically, any food that naturally has an outer shell that can be eaten should be bought organically. The "dirty dozen" items that fall into this category include:

- Nectarines

- Apples

- Peaches

- Pears

- Grapes

- Strawberries

- Bell and hot peppers

- Celery

- Tomatoes

- Cherries

- Spinach

- Kale, collard, and mustard greens

Keep It Simple

A person could become overwhelmed trying to eat organically grown, gluten-free, dairy-free, all-natural, whole foods for every meal and snack. If this is a lot for you because, let's face it, most societies don't center around this kind of eating as a lifestyle, there is still no need to worry. The idea is to try to keep your eating as clean and simple as you can. If you mess up one day, don't beat yourself up about it. If you feel like you can only try cutting out one or two items for a couple of weeks to see how you feel, do that. This experiment in eating should make the most sense for your time and busy life. Again, most people quit diets because they are bored or frustrated with the "all-in" mentality. Instead of thinking this way, get adventurous with new healthy foods that you normally wouldn't choose. Look up recipes (or head to the back of this book!) to see how you can make the most of the flavors in meals. Experiment with the new information you now know because that is one of the ways that you can lead yourself to better digestion and a healthier gut.

Because we're now on a path to cutting certain things out to feel better, the next portion of the book will focus on resetting the process of eating so that you can gain all the benefits from the foods you're eating. This part will also focus on washing out the old and making improvements to the gut for the new healthy items to best serve your body.

Chapter 4:

Tip#2—Detox and Reset

If you don't take care of this, the most magnificent machine that you will ever be given… where are you going to live? –Karyn Calabrese

When was the last time you felt really sweaty and dirty? Maybe you went for a jog on a particularly hot day, and you felt disgusted afterward. Maybe you worked in your garden all afternoon, and your clothes or skin were covered in dirt by the time you finished. Regardless of the scenario, you most likely didn't wait too long to take a nice, warm shower once you were finished with these activities. Typically, humans don't like feeling unclean on the outside.

So, let me now ask you this. Why do people not think of cleaning their internal parts the same as their external ones? When not cared for, our digestive tract can become filled with gross things that we probably won't enjoy thinking about. Because these areas are out of sight and out of mind, we may not give them much thought from day to day. We don't truly know what's going on inside our bodies and may not feel the need to 'clean' ourselves internally as we would externally.

We need to start rethinking this idea. Detoxing our gut not only benefits the digestive tract, but also the mind. The next step toward better gut health is to focus on helpful foods, supplements, and ways to get rid of toxins.

Gut Detoxing the Right Way

When you picture a gut detox, do you imagine a living nightmare of teas, cayenne pepper water, and green juice lunches? Rest assured that this will not be the suggestion in this chapter. A gut detox, or cleanse, is a powerful tool for improved digestion, but it does not need to be painful or hunger-inducing. Typically, when people search for a cleanse online, they'll stumble upon trendy "quick-fixes". While this kind of detoxing may produce some results at first, they typically aren't gentle and won't have a long-lasting impact. They may actually be harmful because they shock the system or don't provide enough nutrients, causing undesirable side-effects.

The suggestions here are designed to help detox the gut and liver by introducing foods, superfoods, supplements, and herbs to the body so that the system can detoxify gently and purposefully. As with anything new, take note of how you feel once you introduce certain things into your body.

A gut detox is beneficial to the entire digestive system. It clears the colon of toxins built up so that nutrients can properly be absorbed, which leads to more regular bowel movements, decreased inflammation, and an overall feeling of wellness. The great news is that it doesn't require any fancy or expensive equipment. In fact, this process can happen without much effort at all.

Supplements and Superfoods

Here's the magical part - Simply by adding and supplementing some of the so-called 'superfoods,' we can naturally detox to improve digestion and add nutrients to the system. Some detox superfoods include apple cider vinegar, spirulina, beets, parsley, cilantro, psyllium husk, and leafy greens (Gut Cleanse: How to Cleanse the Gut to Improve Gut Health?, 2020). Psyllium husk is a gut-cleansing seed that can assist with constipation. Apple cider vinegar, a natural acid, aids in digestion and stimulates the system. Spirulina helps to take toxins and metals out of the system and lowers inflammation. Beets and herbs like parsley and cilantro assist in detoxifying the liver. Leafy greens are excellent in providing minerals, fibers, vitamins, and other nutrients to the system. The beauty of these foods is that most can be added to smoothies, vegetable medleys, or combined into a side dish for easy consumption. A few other important and easy-to-add detox foods are carrots, asparagus, tomatoes, apples, and nuts (Falconer, 2020). The vitamins and minerals quickly take action within the body to ease digestive problems but can also be used to maintain good gut health even when there isn't a problem.

Adding just one or two of these superfoods to salads, gluten-free pasta dishes, or eating them in their whole form for a snack can make a significant difference in the way you feel and live. These foods contribute to an added layer of protection for the body that will continue to work even between meals as well as while you sleep. Bonus! Chapter 9 contains practical recipes that incorporate many superfoods into delicious meals, so consider these meals if you need a starting place.

In addition, garlic, hemp seeds, chia seeds, ginger, avocado, broccoli, and turmeric are great sources to help cleanse the gut and improve digestion. The supplement known as glutathione is an antioxidant that boosts other vitamins and antioxidants in the system, so this one is like a power source to charge the system. This supplement can not only improve digestion but can help with skin, heart, and brain health (Popa, 2019). Magnesium, probiotics, and L-Glutamine are also super helpful supplements.

Other Detoxing Strategies

One of the pieces of advice you've probably heard your whole life is to drink water. Doctors, nutritionists, and the general public are constantly talking about how important water is for the body and how staying hydrated is vital to a person's health. Well, they're right. Drinking water to stay properly hydrated each day is an important way to help the body detox naturally and easily. If you don't currently have a refillable water bottle that you carry around during the day, now is the time to invest in one so you can take water on the go. When you first wake up in the morning, drink some water to give yourself an energy boost. When you go to bed at night, drink a bit of warm water to help you get to sleep. In between these times, set a goal for yourself regarding how many cups you should drink each hour (about two to three). Proper hydration means drinking water frequently throughout the day. The digestive system is stimulated when room temperature water is consumed since this encourages gut movement and breaks up fats in the foods that were consumed (*Is It Better to Drink Cold Water or Room Temperature Water?*, n.d.). Room temperature water helps to boost the metabolism and can even assist with relieving menstrual cramps, which can promote better sleep.

If you find drinking water fairly boring, there are ways to improve the taste and make this liquid more interesting. Try including some natural flavors by adding fruit such as berries, an orange slice, fresh lemon or lime juice, slices of cucumber, or fresh mint leaves. Tongue scraping is another detox method that most wouldn't think is associated with gut health but can actually aid the digestive system. "Tongue scraping can be wonderfully cleansing for your entire body. In fact, your tongue is a direct route to detoxification" (Boghos, 2020). Copper tongue scrapers are available for purchase online, and the process of tongue scraping is quite simple. Before brushing your teeth in the morning, use a tongue scraper to scrape the surface of the tongue, starting at the back of the mouth and moving to the front. Do this several times, rinsing the scraper between each. You'll most likely notice oral hygiene improvements as well as digestive improvements.

Dry brushing also has its benefits. This is the process of using a stiff-bristled brush to remove dry, dead skin to assist with detoxifying the body (*The Truth about Dry Brushing*, 2021). This is particularly helpful to the skin, blood circulation, and the nervous system because it promotes lymph flow and the drainage of toxins. Several YouTube tutorials exist on dry brushing if you're interested in more information on this detoxifying process.

So you may have over-indulged on unhealthy foods or had a bit too much alcohol and you don't feel great. What should you do? There are several methods to help you detox and feel well again. But first, try to remember to take a digestive enzyme before eating things that can cause bloating or irritation to the gut. It's not a catch-all that will magically prevent upset stomachs, but it definitely makes a difference when consuming hard-to-digest items. I know we've been over this already, but I'll say it again—drink water! Drinking warm water with a squeeze of juice from half a lemon can stimulate movement in the digestive tract. Green tea and dandelion root tea also act as effective de-bloaters.

Foods such as bell peppers, garlic, onions, watermelon, cucumbers, grapes, ginger, and berries work as natural diuretics that clean the system. Foods that you may want to avoid if you're feeling bloated or full are grains, dairy, beans, alcohol, and processed foods, as these will trigger more indigestion (Clifford, 2021).

Eating certain foods that are considered prebiotics, such as fruits, nuts, seeds, avocados, and non-starchy vegetables, can also help to counteract any damage from the not-so-healthy stuff. "Prebiotics are a form of dietary fiber that feeds the 'friendly' bacteria in your gut" (Semeco, 2016).

Be sure to include probiotic-rich foods or take a probiotic supplement to assist in healthier digestion. Fermented foods like pickles, sauerkraut, and kimchi, as well as foods like yogurt and sourdough bread, contain probiotics to help balance digestion (Cleveland Clinic, 2020). Try adding foods rich in probiotics as a snack or side dish during mealtime.

Exercise is a natural way to help with digestion if you've eaten a large meal or a meal containing foods that may not make you feel well. To ease digestive trouble, try taking a slow or moderate walk or doing some stretching, especially stretches that gently twist the abdomen. This can promote healthier digestion so that you feel better faster. Next, we will discuss ways to heal and nourish our systems from the inside.

Chapter 5:

Tip#3—Heal and Nourish

You're now on the road to better gut health and understanding some of the foods that will bring out the best performance for your body. You've taken an important and necessary step towards improved digestion, but it takes more than simply changing your diet to feel significantly better. In this chapter, we'll explore ways to restore healthy bacteria and heal the gut lining so that the microbiomes are nourished and protected. While a majority of this protection will come from the foods we ingest, we'll examine additional ways to protect the gut as much as possible through activities that we can include each day. Get ready to heal and feel rejuvenated.

Gut Healing Overview

If you've had days recently where you just feel 'off' and you're not sure why, then you'll most likely benefit from this next part. Taking control of healing your gut has a lot to do with what we choose to put our system through. If our stomach and colon feel any strain from this, we're likely to feel the negative impact of this stress in other areas of our body as well, including our mind. Starting the gut healing process does not need to be a challenging ordeal, it simply needs to be something that you prioritize so that good bacteria can start to work in your system for you to feel better overall. Studies show that over 90% of serotonin, a chemical that sends messages among cells in the body, is produced in the gut (*Study Shows How Serotonin and a*

Popular Anti-Depressant Affect the Gut's Microbiota, 2019). This makes sense when you think about the impact that foods and beverages can have on our moods, emotions, and happiness. If you've ever experienced having a large fried meal or drinking a bit too much alcohol, you've probably felt the impact of these activities on your gut health. Eating or drinking too much may temporarily relieve a desire we have to feel full or satisfied, but this feeling quickly leaves us wanting more. Eating the right foods to promote healthy bacteria helps serotonin send positive messages throughout the body. When we consume foods that are healthier for us, we also feel a sense of satisfaction instead of a deficit.

In addition to certain processed and unhealthy foods, birth control, antibiotics, and certain over the counter painkillers leave the body aching for probiotics in the system because these items will strip away the good bacteria in the gut (Vich Vila et al., 2020). Adding fermented foods to your diet can help restore the good bacteria that certain medications may take away. As mentioned before, try adding yogurt, kefir, kombucha, kimchi, or sauerkraut to your diet to give your body a boost of probiotics. You'll likely find that your digestion improves after consuming any of these foods over a period of time since they help replenish the good bacteria in your gut. Adding these will give your microbiome a fighting chance against any harmful products that may go into your system.

Once you incorporate healthy foods into your diet, it will feel more natural and routine to do so, and you won't feel like you're struggling to replace the foods you once craved. Eating fewer or no processed foods tends to change the way a person thinks about eating in general. You'll probably find that your body and mind are adjusting and that you no longer desire the same foods you once did because your body now feels healthier.

How to Start the Healing Process

To get started, try incorporating some gut superfoods into your system. The three main superfoods that are easy to try today are extra virgin olive oil, spinach, and kefir, a yogurt drink containing healthy bacteria (Hanna, 2021). These foods work to repair and recharge the gut so it's ready to absorb nutrients more effectively. Creating spinach salads with an olive oil-based dressing and adding in some of your favorite veggies is the perfect way to start helping your system.

Stay mindful of the sugar content in some of the items you start incorporating. Kombucha, for example, is a great fermented drink that helps aid digestion, but certain brands can contain high sugar amounts, so be mindful of this and only drink half a bottle at a time. Don't be afraid to try foods you've never had before as you navigate your way through this nutritious adventure. You may discover a food or recipe that you love that could become a new staple in your diet. For example, by adding kimchi or sauerkraut to a veggie sandwich with gluten-free bread, you may discover you enjoy the tangy taste and find that this opens new lunch or dinner options for you. Health food stores carry plenty of alternative options for dairy, meats, and processed foods, so you may want to search your area to find a store that can help you in your quest for good gut health.

A few other foods that are rich in nutrients and will act as prebiotics in your system include sweet potatoes, onions, chickpeas, asparagus, quinoa, and broccoli (Semeco, 2016). The recipes at the end of this book include many of these items, but you can also search for interesting and appealing new recipes for yourself. The idea is to make what you eat interesting, so you won't become bored and want to return to old habits of eating foods that are harder on your system. There are many delicious options for gut health and incorporating a variety of new foods is key! For more information and ideas, peek at Chapter 9.

Activities for Healing the Gut

As mentioned, eating healthy foods is not the only way to heal the gut. In fact, there are methods to heal the gut that don't involve food at all, but these should be combined with a healthy diet. Staying hydrated with plenty of water is one of the best and fastest ways to heal gut microbiomes. Remember to drink water throughout your day by setting timers for yourself as a reminder and drinking glasses of water before each meal so that your food is best absorbed when it passes through.

Try to get the necessary hours of sleep so that your gut is capable of functioning properly. Like me, you'll probably find that if you have difficulty sleeping due to poor gut health, this will improve as your diet changes, so be sure to fully engage in better habits by going to bed earlier and getting enough hours at night. The Sleep Research Society and the American Academy of Sleep Medicine recommend that adults sleep for at least seven hours every night for general health and well-being (*CDC Newsroom*, 2016). Receiving less than this can result in problems with heart disease, obesity, and anxiety, so making every effort to get yourself on a good schedule is important. Make sure to eat meals several hours before you plan to go to bed, and try winding down with soft music, a bath, a book, or other non-electronic methods of relaxation. Stay consistent with your bedtime and sleep routine, as this is one of the best ways to make sure you will get enough rest at night. For adults, getting between seven and nine hours of sleep each night can ensure that they are less susceptible to inflammatory diseases and poor digestive health (MasterHealth Staff, 2022).

In general, lowering stress levels can assist with gut health, but this is often easier said than done. You're most likely a busy person trying to keep yourself afloat throughout the day, which can increase stress on the body. Being a busy person myself, I understand that this is challenging, so look for small opportunities to incorporate moments of stress relief into your day. Taking a short (20–30-minute) walk, watching your favorite show while cooking dinner, or listening to a quick meditation from a downloaded app are ways to improve your mood and make you feel recharged. We'll explore ways that movement and self-care can improve digestion in future chapters, but you can start simply today by getting out in the sunshine for a short walk, breathing in some fresh air, and completing a small deep-breathing exercise. If you're making your health a priority by putting nutritious foods into your body, be sure to not neglect your mind, as the two need to work together on this journey.

Nourishing Supplements for Gut Healing

Not only can healthy foods, water, self-care, rest, and exercise help in keeping our microbiome balanced, but supplements can also play an integral role in healing and maintaining gut health. Both prebiotics and probiotics are efficient ways to help the gastrointestinal tract. Prebiotics and probiotics help feed the good bacteria in the gut so that digestion improves. This can mainly happen by eating the healthy foods we've discussed but can also occur through supplements in the form of pills, powders, or liquids (Lewis, 2020). There are many products out there, so it is helpful to read labels and decide which probiotic may be the most beneficial for you based on your needs.

"L-glutamine is a type of amino acid which has been shown to heal the intestinal wall. It's a key supplement in addressing 'leaky gut' and healing the mucosal lining of the intestines" (Kellman, 2022). This supplement allows particles to break down so they can more easily pass through the digestive tract. This allows the good bacteria to better absorb into the lining of the gut, giving you a better feeling as digestion takes place.

Collagen is a type of protein that we lose as we age. Taking a collagen supplement can help to add this protein back into the system so that it can aid in stomach digestion and heal any damage to the lining of the intestines (Kellman, 2022). Collagen can be consumed in pill form or powder form. I like to add the Vital Proteins brand of collagen powder to my smoothies in the morning, but it can also be added to water, tea, or coffee. With this supplement, it may be necessary to take at least 10g per day to see results, but I find that it helps immensely. Organic bone broth, which can be purchased or homemade, is also a great source of collagen. I will often heat beef or chicken bone broth and sip this throughout the day or have a glass in the evening. Finally, licorice root and marshmallow root are recommended for easing ulcers and repairing intestinal damage. Both can assist in aiding digestion, specifically constipation and heartburn (Cronkleton, 2017). You can find these supplements online or at health food stores.

These foods and supplements are very beneficial to healing the gut and allowing nutrients to digest successfully in the system. Since you now have a better idea of what to add to your diet, in the next parts, we'll detail the methods for optimizing and maintaining good gut health. As with the other methods of improving digestion in this book, consistency is key.

Chapter 6:

Tip#4—Optimize and

Maintain

...our body is an ecosystem. This ecosystem must be maintained... –Ilchi Lee

I hope you are feeling more comfortable experimenting with what feels good for your body on this leg of our journey. If a new or old food does not feel right or upsets your stomach, try something else and take note of how you feel. Again, I do not believe in diets that place a person in a restrictive box. So, I want you to learn as much as possible about your body as you explore what helps you feel better, so if you're ever feeling deprived, something needs to change.

This chapter will center on optimizing digestion and maintaining a healthier gut microbiome and healthy hormones so your body will work at its best. I'm a firm believer that this journey should make the most sense for your needs and lifestyle. Personally, I will sometimes add animal products to my diet, and sometimes I won't. I've learned to gauge how I feel and what my body needs at certain times. I also don't want to feel deprived while eating, so I know that I need to make choices that will satisfy me the most. I encourage you to do this as well. Consider the products that you're purchasing and weigh what you now know. If you can eat high-quality animal products that are grass-fed, organic, and free-range, you will likely notice a positive impact on how you feel after consuming them. Cutting out processed foods will also have a positive impact on your health, but never having a processed meal again may be impossible for some. Perhaps you buy and eat only whole foods at home, then occasionally eat a meal at a restaurant that contains a processed food or two. The key is to start making conscious, mindful choices about your eating so that you get into the habit of understanding what foods will work best for your body.

Tips for Maintaining a Healthy Gut Microbiome

Just as a garden needs tending so that plants can grow, the gut needs some maintenance to ensure that the nutrients entering the body are working to help keep it active and functioning. If you're not already doing so by now, start thinking about meals as your energy source. Food gives you life and it helps you perform for yourself as well as for others. You probably have a good sense of how your body feels when you are sick, so you understand how important it is to care for your body, so it is less likely to shut down. Making a conscious point to add good ingredients to your diet will help you think of your body as the 'bank' that stores and uses these healthy ingredients in a positive way. Like money in this bank, spending all of your time and energy on things that are not useful to you will only lead to negative results. You shouldn't put yourself in a restrictive box when it comes to eating, but you should learn to listen to what your body is telling you about certain foods.

Regularly eating fiber, fermented foods, and as many fresh fruits and vegetables as possible will strengthen your body and can help prevent illness and disease. When planning meals, first consider what main ingredient will help your body the most, then plan your healthy, nutritious meal around this. For example, quinoa is rich in vitamins and protein, so having this as the main ingredient, and then adding some vegetables like roasted sweet potatoes and kale can create a meal that is packed with power and vitamins. When possible, try to make meat the side dish instead of the main focus of the meal. Brighten up your meals by using as many colorful vegetables and fruits as possible. Remember that adding variety to the meals you eat throughout the week will help you feel excited and prevent you from getting bored with your meals. These foods will be working for you long after mealtime is over, so choose ones that you know will provide you with the nourishment that you'll need to work or play through the rest of your day. The buildup of good bacteria will help you to regularly feel good, so if you happen to notice that you have more energy and are more satisfied with the healthier foods instead of feeling hungry an hour after lunch, you'll know why. You're building healthy gut bacteria and your healthy choices will sustain you for long stretches of time.

A helpful idea to practice during your food journey is the 80/20 rule, where you focus on eating healthy ingredients 80% of the time and include the less healthy ones in your diet only 20% of the time (Schetler, 2021). This rule of thumb is achievable for many since it gives a more realistic goal when eating healthier and since it is more concrete to follow. Drink plenty of water as part of the 80% so your system stays hydrated and pushes foods through the digestive tract.

When stress is lower in the body, the gut naturally has an opportunity to feel healthier. I know this sounds easier said than done because stress is difficult to avoid, but when we find opportunities to care for ourselves by taking time to calm our systems down with some deep breathing, short meditation, or a walk in the fresh air, we reset our systems to be more productive and less stressed. When feeling overwhelmed, try taking a few quick moments to step outside and recharge, if only for a short amount of time. A calmer gut is a healthier gut because less stress allows the system to relax and food to pass through in a more productive way. If you're like many people, when you feel stressed, you may notice that your digestive system doesn't feel great either. Taking short breaks throughout the day to help your body relax can do wonders for your brain and gut, so make time for these breaks and you will most likely notice a difference in your digestion.

The Gut Health Cheat Sheet

Because variety will help you stay on track and interested in healthier foods, it's important to choose and add a wide range of plant-based foods into the eating rotation. To do this, try choosing between 10–20 plant-based items each week that you can incorporate into meals at home. This will give you a base to work from and will keep you motivated because of the variety. It won't feel like you're depriving yourself when you have so many items to choose from. Make a list of your favorites and see how many you can come up with. Then add to this list by researching additional plant-based foods that you may learn to love. Or, if you're short on time, use the cheat sheet below to choose items that sound interesting to you while you mix and match your way to better meal planning.

Leafy Greens	Fruits	Meat, Fish, and Eggs (add sparingly)	Healthy Oils, Fats, and Broth
• spinach • kale • arugula • cabbage • romaine lettuce • bok choy • swiss chard	• berries • apple • oranges • mango • banana • kiwi • papaya • lemon • lime	• free-range, organic chicken or turkey • grass-fed, organic beef • free-range eggs • salmon • tuna	• avocado • extra virgin olive oil • coconut oil • sesame oil • flaxseed oil • bone broth (organic, grass-fed, free range)
Root Vegetables	**Sprouts, Seeds, and Nuts**	**Fermented Foods**	**Grains**
• sweet potatoes • potatoes • carrots • squash • jicama • beets	• broccoli • alfalfa • mung bean • pumpkin seeds • chia • flaxseed • cashews • almonds	• kefir • kimchi • probiotic yogurt • sauerkraut • tempeh • miso • kombucha	• quinoa • wild rice • basmati rice • steel cut oats • gluten-free oats • spelt • brown rice

This menu is fine for when you're cooking at home, but what happens when you want to eat out at a restaurant? It becomes trickier for many people when they go out to eat because we tend to splurge on meals that we wouldn't usually have at home or make for ourselves. Sometimes splurging is alright within reason, but it's necessary to keep our goal in mind: to consistently have better gut health. One processed item at a restaurant may not mess with your digestive system much, but three or four might. Remember that we're building healthy gut health habits so that you're able to have good bacteria in your system so that these microbiomes will assist in the fight against any bad bacteria. It's also important to continue to make mindful food choices even when all the items on a menu look tempting.

Now, how does one stick to their healthy eating habits when going out to eat? One of the best ways is to be the one that chooses the restaurant. If you know of one that serves more plant-based options or has an extensive menu including a variety of vegetables, suggest this as the restaurant you attend. If you're unable to make the final decision on where you go, be sure to check the menu in advance to make a healthy plan for yourself. Remember to do this when you're not hungry so you aren't tempted by every food item on the menu. Another helpful tip is to eat a small, healthy snack before you go so that you don't want to order everything you see and can be mindful when choosing. Staying conscious of the decisions you're making will give you more control of how your digestive system will react.

At home or while dining out, remind yourself of how you want to feel after you eat a meal. You've probably experienced some tough times in the past with stomach issues after consuming foods that were difficult for your body to digest, and you want to avoid feeling this way again. At restaurants, be sure to look for the leafy greens on the menu first. Depending on the restaurant, you can most likely find at least one leafy green and ask for modifications if it comes with additional processed fats, oils, dairy, or gluten. Next, look for other veggies, like carrots, sweet potatoes, or broccoli. Sometimes these items may be soaked in butter or oil, so ask questions to find out if you can have them prepared differently. I know this is difficult, and other people may give you the side eye, but similar to an allergy, if you explain that you have dietary restrictions, most restaurants tend to accommodate their customers. Check the sides on the menu, as this section tends to contain many of the vegetables that are served with meals, and you could order several of these or ask for a side dish with a salad. Finally, check for proteins as there may be some slightly healthier options like a veggie burger or a filet of salmon. Just in case you decide to splurge on dairy or gluten options, you may want to take some digestive enzymes with your meal if you suspect that it may upset your stomach. Restaurants can provide us with opportunities to eat foods we wouldn't normally make for ourselves, but when going out to eat, keep in mind the progress you've made with your gut health and continue to make the healthiest choices possible so that you don't undo what you've started.

Tips for Mindful Eating

While factoring in what foods may work best for your personal meal plan, it's important to know yourself. What kinds of ingredients do you personally need to buy to keep at home and eat? If you live with others, these may be different from the kinds of meals that your roommates or family members are eating, although they don't have to be. No matter what, keep in mind what is best for you and slow down to mindfully connect with food and improve your eating habits.

Choose things that will act as fuel for your body. This doesn't mean that they can't taste good. Of course, they can, but make a choice to decide on the right foods and recipes that will nourish and replenish your energy. In your search for healthy items that you will love; find ones that will feel satisfying and keep you full longer, as well as ones that you actually want to eat. If you try a food and find that you don't like it, try preparing it differently or try something else altogether. When you find something you love, add it to a list of ingredients or recipes that you can place in rotation when you want something that you already know is delicious and gratifying.

When you choose to mindfully eat, you can feel powerful because you are the one in control. Remind yourself that it's okay to feel hungry and use the opportunity to gauge just how hungry you are or if you are actually hungry at all. For many, we eat out of boredom or stress, so knowing this about ourselves can help us understand our own habits and patterns so we can change the cycle. Really consider what you will have and how much you will need to feel satisfied. Chew each bite slowly so that you can actually taste the foods you've chosen and prepared. Sit in a chair at a table instead of while you rush around the house or drive somewhere. The bottom line is to take your time to appreciate what is in front of you and think about what you're doing. This not only aids in digestion but also helps you to know when you're satisfied so that you don't overeat and feel sick. Drink water before and after to bookend the meal and to help carry it properly through your digestive tract.

Whether you eat meals alone or with other people, make it an event instead of scarfing down the food as fast as you can. If you're eating a meal with company, take deep breaths between bites and have a conversation with others. When you slow down, your stomach will thank you later by not having to work as hard to break up your food.

Again, always eat when you are hungry. If you have a plan in mind with some staple snacks or meals that you like, this will help during times when your stomach actually feels hungry. Eat throughout your day so you don't deprive yourself of opportunities to eat and then overindulge by mistake. This will cause more irritation to the gut as it tries to comprehend what has hit it so quickly. When it's mealtime or snack time, engage the senses by appreciating the look, smell, feel, and taste of the foods that you're consuming. Put any electronic devices to the side for the mealtime, as you should engage fully in this experience to get the most out of it. Appreciate the nutrients that will strengthen your body and mind and know that the foods you put in now will continue to work to make you healthier and more energized long after you eat them. This may sound silly but taking the time to honor the foods you have and are able to eat will allow you to be more mindful about showing gratitude toward everyday items that you are fortunate enough to have in your life. Try this today, right now even, by making yourself a snack, then sitting and appreciating everything about the food that you've just prepared. Consider what you love about it and enjoy the process.

The steps ahead will give you an opportunity to optimize gut and hormone health through exercise and movement. This is an important part of gut health that often gets ignored. Learning about this next step will offer gradual, gentle improvements so that exercise can be a part of your life if it isn't already. If it is, you will have a chance to try moving more mindfully as you engage your body in healthy activities.

Chapter 7:

Tip#5—Move Your Body

Those who think they have no time for bodily exercise will sooner or later have to find time for illness. –Edward Stanley

If you've ever been to an intense cardio fitness class or worked with a personal trainer, you've probably experienced feelings of panic as you work to keep up with a quick pace. Phrases like "one more rep" or "no pain, no gain" may have been yelled in your direction as you struggle to breathe and wipe the sweat off your face. You may have secretly thought to yourself, "I'm so stressed out from exercising. How is this possibly doing my body any good?" If you've ever thought this way, you're not so far off. Many people get the impression that when it comes to exercise, they need to push themselves as hard as humanly possible to get any results. Similar to intense dieting, when we do this to our bodies, we tend to burn out quickly and give up before any real progress can be made. Imagine what this kind of stress and intensity is doing to your gut as well. If you feel stressed and overwhelmed by the mere thought of a workout, your brain is going to send messages to your digestive system to feel tense and stressed about it as well. For actual results to happen, we need to rethink our old ways of exercising and start focusing on what is best for our bodies.

My struggle with exercise and weight loss began like so many other people's. I wanted to lose some weight to get healthier, so I tried intensely working out for hours at a time, longing for results. I didn't see them. After pushing myself too hard, I found myself so exhausted, both physically and mentally, that I would simply collapse at the end of each day. I felt like I had no time to recharge my brain with something gentle and healthy because, I thought, if I was doing slow exercise, I wasn't maximizing the results I could get by doing intense workouts instead. Everything felt difficult and forced with my exercise routine because that's the way I thought it needed to be. I checked my weight on the scales each morning and, nothing. I was not seeing results, and on top of this, I was feeling worse because my mind and stomach were stressed from the intense workouts I was putting my body through. I knew this was not a sustainable way to live, but I wasn't sure what exercise routine I should follow instead.

I decided I needed to listen to my body more and make decisions based on what felt manageable. For me, this meant that instead of running on a treadmill as fast as I could, I would take a moderately-paced walk outside each day for at least 30 minutes. Instead of getting yelled at to get moving in a cardio class at the gym, I would do 10 to 15 minutes of stretching and toning at home each morning when I first woke. This felt right for me and, after a couple of weeks of feeling more relaxed with my workouts, I started seeing results. I surprised myself with this. The weight that I was trying to lose seemed to come off easily, almost effortlessly. My digestion and mental clarity improved as well. I felt more relaxed and able to make better choices with my eating habits because I wasn't starving after workouts like I was before. I felt like I had finally made a breakthrough and actually looked forward to the quiet time that I would allow myself to have while exercising. It became my moment of Zen.

I want to stress here that my story is just one example of what worked for me. I saw a need to change the structure of how I was working out, and I made that accommodation for myself. What I want you to remember is that everyone's path will be different. If you find that an intense workout is fun or energizing for you and you look forward to it, you don't need to stop doing this for yourself simply because I'm saying this wasn't for me. Personalize your journey on what works best for you. Allow for changes and adjustments to be made along the way. Explore new movements and workouts to see what feels right. You will most likely find that when you're happy with the activities that you're doing, your body will react in a way that feels calm and relaxed. This will naturally help keep the gut calm and relaxed as well.

Get in the Gut Health Mindset

If you've struggled to find the motivation to exercise in the past, it may be time to redefine the way you think of "working out." This image no longer needs to be associated with intensity and sweating. Instead of thinking, "Ugh, I have to work out," change your mindset to "Yay, I GET to work out." I know, I know, this sounds a bit too optimistic, but think about this idea for a moment. If you're capable of functional body movement in any way, be grateful for this. Your body is an amazingly powerful mechanism that can do much more than you think. Start to listen to it and embrace what it can do. Remember that nothing has to be perfect about your workout, and if you don't like one exercise, you can try something else. Part of having and maintaining a healthy gut mindset is to recognize that it's fine to rest and that it's healthy to take breaks. Nothing needs to feel forced because this feeling may lead to stress. In fact, a person who works out intensely for several days a week may be triggering their cortisol, or stress hormone, to continue feeling elevated, which will lead to even more stress (Kassel, 2018). The key is to mix up your workout, so it feels right for you and to remember to put your feelings first when listening to your body.

Exercising for Your Gut Health

If you are trying to lose weight, the foods you eat will play a large role in this. In fact, when it comes to weight loss, the things we ingest seem to have more of an impact than physical activity. By watching what we eat and maintaining steady, healthy eating habits, a person can have more success in losing weight than they could with exercise alone (Roth, 2018). While we've covered some of the major ways to improve gut health with foods, it's also important to find a balance between eating and exercise so that we can keep moving to improve the microbiome even more.

With a routine of exercise, we are able to prevent disease and common illnesses as well as ease inflammation in the gut (Kozmor, n.d.). When our digestive tract has healthy, diverse bacteria in it from the foods we eat, it automatically works better for us, resulting in more energy. If we've already been practicing good gut health by adding the right nutrients, exercise is like the icing on the gluten-free cake. It will only enhance the work we've already put into our healthy eating plan.

The good news is that exercise doesn't need to be strenuous or challenging; it just needs to happen consistently. Even if you've never exercised a day in your life, you can start moving in small ways so that you feel a positive change. Over time, the movement leads to a reduction in inflammation and intestinal permeability and improves body composition (Clauss et al., 2021). Walking, swimming, biking, and even gentle yoga or stretching all count toward physical activity that will help us improve the way we feel.

Since exercise tends to prevent illness and promote energy, you'll probably find that you feel like you're able to do more activities as time passes and you continue your routine. You'll notice that foods may digest better and that your hormone levels feel more regulated throughout the day. In addition, exercise helps with the production of Vitamin B and K, two essential vitamins used in the digestive process (*5 Exercises That Aid in Optimal Digestive Health - ADH*, 2022). As we age, we tend to lose mobility, so even gentle, consistent movements during the day can help to keep us active as we get older.

Starting and Maintaining an Exercise Routine

It's difficult to know what will feel right for each individual, so test the waters with exercise and see what makes you happy. If exercising is new to you, it's especially important to make a point of scheduling it in your day, just as you would schedule an important event or meeting. Decide what time of day is going to work best for you so that you won't lose motivation. I like to start my morning with exercise because then I know that I'll make it a priority. Plus, it is a mood booster and gives me some great energy to continue functioning throughout my day. By introducing a short workout to your schedule, you will begin to feel more energized too. Simply getting outside for a 20–30-minute walk will give you some mental clarity and give your metabolism a boost. Aim for about 5,000 to 10,000 steps a day to help your body and digestive system feel healthier.

If the thought of even gentle exercise makes you groan, try finding a task that can take your mind away from the part that feels difficult. For example, if you like to read, listen to a downloaded book on your phone as you walk. Listening to books, podcasts, or music is a great way to pass the time while exercising. Call a friend and talk to them while you walk, or even better, invite them along to have a workout buddy.

You already know that getting some daily fresh air is helpful, but what if you live in an area that experiences fluctuating seasons, making it difficult to exercise in extreme cold or heat? Well, try getting outside anyway since this truly will bring stress levels down throughout your day. Bundle up if it's cold or snowing; take an umbrella if it's raining; wear sunscreen if it's hot; but make a point to get outside to experience the outdoors, even if you're only there for a few minutes. The effort you make to do this will help blood flow throughout your body and will assist your lymphatic system in removing toxins.

Remember to start small as you don't want to burn out with your effort to include working out in your schedule. If nothing else, find creative ways to get moving, like parking your car further away from your destination or taking the stairs instead of an elevator. If you have a job that keeps you busy and away from the gym, there are still several kinds of exercises you can include during your day to benefit your gut health. These include movements that you can even complete while on a break at work. Try gentle yoga, sit-ups, or crunches, and pelvic floor exercises, which can all be accomplished in a small space. If you have a coworker who would be interested in taking a walk during lunch, schedule this time into your day and bring walking shoes to work. Any of these suggested activities will help in the digestive process and bring you a sense of relief throughout the week, so save yourself some time each day to participate in some physical activities.

Even striking some yoga poses while you sit in a chair at work can benefit your system. There are plenty of chair yoga videos that exist, so research one that you may find fun. If you have a bit of private space in an office, you may want to consider bringing a yoga mat or a towel to stretch or do a few sit-ups in between meetings and emails. Introducing this into your day can provide a nice break and can give you an opportunity to clear your mind for a few moments as well.

For women, even a brief workout during the day can assist with more balanced hormone levels and less painful menstrual cycles. If you typically get a tired, achy, or 'off' feeling as a result of your menstrual cycle, stretching and movement can naturally alleviate these feelings to some degree. Lower back pain is often associated with a painful cycle, and since this area is near the stomach and colon, doing some gentle twisting stretches may help to clear some of the stress and pain from these areas.

Do What You Can

On certain days, you may only have a few minutes to stretch or move actively, and this is perfectly okay. The idea is to do what you can, when you can, and where you can, so never beat yourself up for not having enough time for a workout; just try again to incorporate exercise the next day. If you realize at the end of your day that you missed finding a time to exercise, there are a few gentle stretches that you can try before bedtime to help calm your nervous system, body, and mind.

While there are many relaxing stretches and yoga videos online, I'm going to share a few of my personal favorites that are specifically for digestive health. For a soothing stretch before bedtime, find a clear area along a wall and try lying on your back while placing your legs up the wall. I know this one sounds difficult, but if you are able to sit on the floor and get up afterward, you have the mobility and skills necessary to complete this. Not only does this pose allow you to rest for a moment, but it also encourages blood flow throughout your system, causing an overall feeling of relaxation. This supports the adrenal glands and helps if your legs, ankles, or feet become swollen throughout the day due to standing in one place or sitting at a desk.

Another amazing stretch comes from lying on your back and bringing the right leg in, then moving it across your body, causing a twist at your waist. Stretch both arms out to the side and turn your neck so you are looking away from the direction of the leg that's crossed over the body. Hold the stretch for at least 20 seconds, then repeat this on the opposite side. This is a natural way to 'wring' out the digestive organs so that any gas or bloating is relieved and the intestinal tract can keep moving.

The yoga favorites that I also love incorporating into my day are cat-cow stretch, crocodile pose, and knees to chest. The cat-cow stretch is a simple one that leaves you feeling more refreshed and energetic. If you can sit on the floor, gently and slowly move so that you are on your hands and knees. Then, just like a cat, round your spine as if something is pulling the center of your back to the ceiling. Drop your head as your spine rounds. Exhale while doing this stretch. Then, do the opposite by lowering the belly and spine and looking upwards while inhaling. Do this one as slowly as you can to get the full relaxation benefits. This will get the blood flowing and the digestive tract working, so it's a great one to start the day with. The crocodile pose is a powerful one that can relax muscles and recharge the body and brain. While lying on your stomach, fold your arms and place them under your forehead so your head has a place to rest. Slowly inhale and exhale and feel your stomach move out and in on the floor under you. This pose stimulates the connective tissue in the stomach so food can move properly through the system (Hopes, 2022). Finally, the simple act of lying on your back and pulling one knee at a time to your chest can go a long way. This stretch also assists with any bloating or gas in the system but is done mindfully to massage the internal organs. Though done in a mild manner, you may feel that you have more energy once you finish completing these exercises, so they truly can provide a surge of vitality if you feel sluggish.

Diaphragmatic breathing is an additional way to calm the nervous system and reduce stress levels. This kind of breathing can allow for full, gentle breaths so that intestinal organs are massaged, and any pain is reduced (Hopes, 2022). This practice is done by sitting tall and placing a hand or hands on the stomach, then slowly breathing in and out for five to ten minutes. Imagine the air flowing in and out of the system as you breathe and notice your hands moving out and then in on your stomach. Doing this before bed or in any moments of stress throughout the day ensures that your body calms itself so it can be more present and comfortable.

If you've noticed the trend of taking care of yourself in the chapters so far, this is not accidental. The ways that you choose to be kind to yourself influence the way that you will act and feel. When your body and mind are relaxed, it is much easier for your stomach to digest and your gut health to improve. Next, we'll look at ways to ensure that you are caring for yourself with simple ideas that you can add to your daily schedule to help you feel relaxed. The correlation between mental health and gut health is closely linked, and methods to reduce stress can have a large impact on the way we feel internally, so that we can feel great externally.

Chapter 8:

Tip#6—Practice Self-Care

Take care of your mind, your body will thank you. Take care of your body, your mind will thank you. –Debbie Hampton

As we wind down our exploration of gut health, let's keep our minds at the forefront of this ongoing discussion as the mind and gut work in tandem while we work, play, and sleep. Stress is a part of life, but each time we push our gut health aside because it's harder to prepare a healthy meal or because we don't feel like exercising, we short-change ourselves of an opportunity. By doing this, we take away a chance to feel less stressed and anxious. We don't let our stomach feel its best or allow ourselves to get enough sleep at night. Ultimately, we wear our systems out when we are so busy that we forget to take time to rest and relax.

Since it's said that the gut is our second brain, we need to acknowledge and address the fact that stress and anxiety will impact the way we feel physically. Even if we were to eat hundreds of vegetables and fruits a day, if our mind doesn't feel healthy, our body won't either. Once we recognize that an overtaxed mind and body can lead to an overtaxed gut, we can start to do something about this. Consistency in caring for ourselves each day is a key piece in creating a routine that we can maintain.

If you are still unsure if the brain has that much control over the gut, let's examine the science behind this. "The brain has a direct effect on your gastrointestinal system because they are intimately connected by your Vagus Nerve—the longest cranial nerve in your body that travels from the brainstem to the lowest part of your intestines" (*Mindset Can Directly Affect Your Digestive System*, 2018). This line of communication sends messages back and forth and, if your stomach is upset, it sends that message back to the brain, causing the brain to stress as well. Likewise, if you are stressed, worried, or afraid of something, this message travels back to the stomach and, ultimately, the entire gastrointestinal system. This is powerful information for us as it demonstrates just how important it is to take care of ourselves.

When problems with the digestive tract are ongoing, the mind can never truly feel relaxed or at rest. Chronic gastrointestinal issues can lead to feelings of depression. The more anxious or depressed an individual feels, the more cortisol, or the stress hormone, gets continuously released into the system, only making matters worse. The lining of the gut can become damaged because of this constant stress, so it's an ongoing and vicious cycle.

In this chapter, we'll work toward stress reduction and management so that our gut health improves. As always, feel free to apply the topics presented so they work best for your lifestyle and needs. Pick ideas that resonate with you and try implementing them into your routine, as this is the best way to create a habit for yourself. I also recommend trying new self-care techniques that you've never tried before, as you may discover something that you love.

While the techniques found in this chapter are gentle and mindful approaches to reducing stress, they may not act as a complete end to the stress cycle a person experiences. With that said, it is also worth examining counseling or cognitive therapy to receive help if you feel that you are doing everything you can to relax, but you still feel an overwhelming amount of stress. "Some patients with functional GI conditions might improve with therapy to reduce stress or treat anxiety or depression.

Multiple studies have found that psychologically based approaches lead to greater improvement in digestive symptoms compared with only conventional medical treatment" (Harvard Health Publishing, 2019). There are many individuals that can assist in the area of depression and anxiety, so if you feel that an independent practice of self-care is not enough, try researching what is available in your area for more information on counseling or therapy near you.

Mental and Gut Health United

Scientists refer to the brain-gut connection as the enteric nervous system, or ENS, which is powerful since it's made up of more than 100 million nerve cells within the gastrointestinal tract (*The Brain-Gut Connection*, 2019). This system aids in the way information travels through the digestive tract and can trigger emotions. When we feel happy, digestion becomes easier, but when we feel unsettled or stressed, our ENS tells the stomach to feel this sensation as well, leaving us with an upset stomach or other symptoms of intestinal distress. While important advances have been made to understand the impact of the ENS on gut health and the ways that the brain and digestive tract are linked, researchers still need more information to understand the link even better. There could be any number of factors impacting gut health today, from modern digital devices to processed foods, so it's vital for individuals who struggle with digestive problems to stay as well-informed as possible with ongoing findings.

Sleep and Self-Care

Because we understand that the mind and gut have a connection that impacts the way we feel, it's easy to see that this connection would impact our sleep patterns as well. Interrupted sleep is common among people who experience stress, so it's especially important to practice stress relieving exercises to calm the mind and body so that the quality of your sleep improves. Stress can specifically impact disorders like insomnia and sleep apnea (Breus, 2022). Practicing better habits can significantly improve rest cycles, so if you do feel that you struggle to fall asleep or stay asleep, there are several practices that you can include in your daily routine.

The first is to ditch the digital devices several hours before bedtime. This one is difficult because many people tend to check emails, send text messages, or watch television shows while in bed. This habit needs to change if you want to fall asleep faster and get a better night's rest. If you feel like you're addicted to your phone and must have it before bed, try simply listening to soft instrumental music or a quiet meditation. Remember to avoid strenuous, stimulating activities two to three hours before bedtime so that you give your body and mind the proper time to unwind. Keep a consistent schedule by going to bed around the same time each night and waking up around the same time each morning. If it helps, set a reminder on your phone to help you start unwinding each evening in preparation for sleep. The main strategy when trying to change a poor bedtime routine is to make your environment comfortable so you can settle your mind and digestive system. Deep breathing, gentle stretching, or reading a book are all excellent ways to clear the mind of that day's events and get into a relaxing state.

Use soft lighting in the evening so your eyes and brain start to calm and get ready for the night. Avoiding caffeine late in the day and alcohol in the evening will also assist with this process. The stimulants in caffeine and the chemicals in alcohol interrupt our sleep cycle, so even if we fall asleep quickly after drinking these products, we will most likely not remain this way for long. Our bodies need time to process and break down the ingredients in either substance, so it's best to leave a long stretch of time, four to five hours, before going to bed after consuming either.

Stress Relievers

If you suffer from digestive problems, you are probably aware of how stress can impact the way you feel. If you're busy and bouncing from one activity to the next all day, it's almost impossible to find adequate time to relieve that stress. You've already learned several methods that help to let the stressful feelings release from your system, such as stretching and walking, but it's worth discussing other forms of relief so that you're armed with a bank of strategies to pull from when you're particularly overwhelmed.

Since you may not be able to control the moments when you're feeling the most stressed, make a list of ideas on your phone or on paper of the best ways for you to relax. Find methods that are the most appealing to you, then be ready to choose one item from this list when you feel overwhelmed. Even better, find the time to save moments in the day to choose at least one item from your list and complete this activity *before* you feel stressed. I know, this seems like a novel idea, but doing this can prevent you from feeling out of control when those stressful moments hit. You'll be armed with relaxation techniques to calm you against the feelings that can cause gut health problems.

Guided Imagery

If you've never tried guided imagery for relaxation, this should definitely go into your bag of tricks as it is one of the best forms of calming yourself down on a particularly stressful day. Guided imagery "can involve imagining yourself being in your 'happy place'—maybe picturing yourself sitting on a beach, listening to the waves, smelling the ocean, and feeling the warm sand underneath you" (Scott, 2021). It's the perfect solution because it can be done anywhere and at any time. If you are able to get to a somewhat quiet space, even a bathroom stall, for a few minutes, close your eyes and imagine yourself in a location of your choosing. Start to picture your whole-body relaxing, from the top of your head to the tips of your toes. Even a few minutes of doing this will help you calm and relax your mind, so it's worth a try. In addition, there are many guided imagery apps that you can download if you need someone else's help to talk you through a peaceful scenario. This is an amazing and powerful tool for the mind as it gives us a space to simply walk through a relaxation of our bodies. It relieves stress almost immediately, and if you're prone to panic attacks like I was, it is a wonderful practice to have at the ready. Having calming thoughts and words go a long way, and having a regular guided practice set in your schedule is a way to remind yourself that you know how to instantly calm the body when you need to.

Walking to Calm Worries

We've talked about the ways that simply walking outdoors can allow you to get some exercise and some fresh air to feel calmer and energized, but now let's discuss the power of this in connection with your brain. This kind of gentle exercise releases endorphins in our brains that have a powerful positive impact on our mental health (Anderer, 2021). Each time we get moving outdoors, we give ourselves a small adventure, which is like an exciting gift for our brain. We can see, hear, smell, and touch new things. The location and time of our experience are in our control, so if your walk ever starts to feel too boring, change it up and try going somewhere different. The stimulation that your brain receives from this will reward your mind and body with a feeling of success and accomplishment. Get out today for a short stroll and see how this impacts your mental health. Go on! This chapter will be here when you return!

The Power of Touch

This next method of stress relief sounds simple, but it has one of the most amazing impacts on our psyche. Hugging another person can allow our bodies to feel a calmness and release that instantly makes us feel happier. "When you hug someone, oxytocin (also known as the 'cuddle hormone') is released. Oxytocin is associated with higher levels of happiness and lower levels of stress" (Scott, 2021). This healing power of touch allows our brain to release stress and take a momentary break from worry. Try this with a loved one soon and feel the benefits that it offers.

Aromatherapy

Have you ever walked into a store and immediately had a sense of calm wash over you because it smelled like a fall breeze, freshly baked cookies, or a pine forest? Our sense of smell has a powerful effect on our mood and demeanor. Using aromatherapy to calm the body through the sense of smell is an easy way to set the tone for the day. The key to this is to find a scent that you love and use it to make you feel more relaxed. Adding a candle, body lotion, or some incense to your space can impact the way you feel and process information so that you can chill out while staying productive and focused.

Relaxation in Art and Music

Somehow, adults forget about taking time to connect with their inner child and participate in activities that will appease their artistic side. If you haven't colored, painted, or made some art in years, it's time to bust out a box of crayons. "Research consistently shows that coloring can have a meditative effect. One study found that anxiety levels declined in people who were coloring complex geometric patterns, making it a perfect outlet for stress reduction" (Scott, 2021). Adult coloring books have gained popularity, and this continues to prove to be a relaxing method for calming the system. Listening to relaxing music throughout the day also influences our overall mood. This is an easy stress reliever to add to your day during a walk or while you work, so try to find some time for it and pay attention to how it makes you feel because, most likely, you'll become more calm and at ease through the power of music.

Chocolate (Yes, Chocolate!)

This next bit of information will come as exciting news for any chocoholics out there. Researchers studied the impact of a person eating one average-sized dark chocolate bar every day for two weeks and found that this reduced the stress hormone, cortisol, as well as the "fight-or-flight" hormone, catecholamines, in highly stressed people (Warner, 2009). Of course, the key to this technique is to not go overboard with eating chocolate, but rather, to allow yourself to indulge in a small amount of dark chocolate as a treat when you're feeling overwhelmed. This method of release is not likely to have a negative impact on the digestive system if you have worked to build and practice good gut health throughout the rest of the day, but as with everything, use your best judgment if chocolate has made your digestive system feel sick previously.

Calming the Nerves from Within

In working toward stress relief, it's important to utilize the benefits of free and easy techniques that you have access to throughout the day. This includes making time for yourself to practice calming exercises that will help your brain and body. If you are on a tight schedule, meditation, deep breathing exercises, and journaling are simple, yet effective, methods of relaxation that take only a few minutes. Choose a method and add it to your upcoming week to start feeling the benefits of clarity and awareness.

Mindful Meditation

One overlooked area that can improve mental health, as well as gut health, is making meditation part of a daily routine. Meditating for even five to ten minutes is a powerful way to decrease anxiety and create feelings of peace and happiness in oneself. Meditation can be personalized so that it fits your comfort level and lifestyle as well. If you are not keen on crossing your legs on the floor, try simply sitting in a chair and closing your eyes for a few minutes to get some inner peace. Saying a positive affirmation or mantra to yourself, such as "I am strong" or "I am healthy," can add a boost of confidence and motivation to your day. There are many guided meditation apps to use if you feel you need a voice to help you in this process, so don't be afraid to give these a try. Also, try not to put pressure on yourself to completely zone out. Simply making time to sit and be still for a few moments is enough to lower your cortisol level and help balance hormones, even if your mind wanders while trying to meditate. Find a practice that works for you and make time for it. When your practice becomes a consistent part of your day, you'll surprise yourself with an improved mood and an overall sense of well-being, which is sure to have great effects on your digestive system.

Deep Breathing

Practicing deep breathing techniques when you're stressed has a quick, calming effect and can be done anywhere or at any time of the day. This is a powerful tool to have in your stress-relieving arsenal since it requires no equipment and almost instantly calms the nerves. A great technique is box breathing, which involves breathing in for a count of four, holding the breath for a count of four, then breathing out for a count of four, holding for a count of four, and continuing to repeat the cycle (Scott, 2020). This kind of breathing is a fast way to calm the system and reset the mind.

Another strategy to try is the alternate nostril breathing technique, which simply means breathing in through one nostril while holding the other nostril closed with your thumb, then switching to closing the other nostril and breathing out of the other side, repeating and switching on both sides for five to ten cycles (*What to Know about Alternate-Nostril Breathing*, n.d.). Decide on a technique that feels good to you and work to incorporate it for a brief amount of time each day. These techniques are quick and simple, so they can easily fit into a busy lifestyle. Each time you practice a breathing exercise, notice the relief and relaxation you feel after.

Journaling for Mental Health

If you've tried incorporating meditative and breathing practices into your day, journaling can be an additional way to bring calmness to your life. While journaling can stimulate the mind, it can also provide a space for any and every thought you are having. This helps our mind to relax since it is a cathartic way to release our thoughts and feelings. Our writing doesn't even need to make sense as we do it, it simply needs to keep flowing so we can get these thoughts on paper. Journaling can also be an amazing way to capture hopes and goals on paper so that we have a chance to visualize what it is that we want in life, then manifest it into reality. Try setting a timer and allowing yourself an uninterrupted 10 or 15 minutes to simply write so you can see what flows from your brain. This is a great practice for stimulating the mind as well, so try it without placing pressure on yourself to come up with something that makes sense or is even written well. Just let the words dump out onto the page. You can read it back to yourself at the end or not. Either way, you will find this a grounding, peaceful, safe space to generate real thoughts.

If you find yourself feeling stuck when getting started with journaling, try researching a prompt that you would like to respond to. There are hundreds of great ones that exist online and can help you get your pen writing. You can even simply choose an affirming statement like "I am calm" and write it over and over again for five to ten minutes to simply get into the habit of grounding and calming yourself for a period of time each day.

One of my personal favorite journaling techniques is to write about what my future will look like. I give myself time to reflect on what I would like to accomplish and how I want to feel as a result of my progress. This gives me a sense of appreciation for the focus that I am working toward my goals. I can also take moments to appreciate the goals that I've already accomplished. With this kind of journaling, it may be important to read it back to yourself occasionally, to see how you're progressing or to make any adjustments to your goals. I'd suggest splurging on a nice hardcover, lined-paper journal and a fancy pen for yourself so that the thought of writing for a few minutes daily will excite you instead of overwhelming you. Journaling can be a wonderfully calming practice but find ways that work for you so that you will want to incorporate this into your life.

Herbs, Tinctures, and Supplements

In addition to the techniques in this chapter, herbs, tinctures, and supplements can help ease stress naturally. You may have heard of the benefits of lavender, for example, which is a plant said to provide calming relief to the nervous system. Many people are drawn to this relaxing scent and purchase lavender essential oils for its soothing fragrance. Try placing a small drop of oil on your pillow to settle your mind at night.

Lemon balm is an herb that is ingested to help the nervous and digestive systems. This herb "was used as far back as the Middle Ages to reduce stress and anxiety, promote sleep, improve appetite, and ease pain and discomfort from indigestion (including gas and bloating, as well as colic)" (*Lemon Balm Information | Mount Sinai - New York*, n.d.). People today still report the benefits they feel from this herb after struggling with insomnia, anxiety, or an upset stomach.

Sometimes bitters are used to create interesting cocktails, but many people use them for anxiety and digestive relief as well. Typically, bitters come in the form of a tincture, and a few drops of the liquid can be placed in a drink or directly on the tongue. The bitter agents in bitters, like wormwood, artichoke leaf, or dandelion root, have a calming effect and can be incorporated into a self-care routine (La Forge, 2021).

Rhodiola Rosea is yet another herb that promotes anxiety relief, treats fatigue, and possibly protects against illness. This herb comes in capsule or tincture form and is said to have benefits for enhancing brain function and supporting the adrenal gland so that stress is lowered (Kubala, 2021).

Herbal tea is a tried-and-true natural defense against anxiety and stress. Teas such as chamomile, peppermint, and valerian soothe and calm the system and act as a helper for digestion (Braun & Caplan, 2021). Choose organic herbal teas so that you can get the best benefits from the herbs without ingesting pesticides. For those struggling with irritable bowel syndrome (IBS), colitis, or Crohn's disease, herbal teas can add soothing relief to your digestive system throughout the day.

Ashwagandha and reishi mushroom powder, capsules, or tea add a sense of calm to the body so that sleep and anxiety relief can happen. In a 2019 study, ashwagandha extract was found to significantly help decrease mental stress in participants compared to individuals who took a placebo (Parch, 2020). Reishi mushrooms are said to boost the immune system and prevent fatigue (Tinsley, 2018). These findings may prove to help many in their struggles with anxious feelings and provide a more natural form of relief. I've found that my favorite brands for mushroom supplements are Four Sigmatic and RealMushrooms, both of which can be purchased online.

In searching for what relief may be right for you, consider any current medications you are on and speak with your doctor about drug interactions or even the possibility of alternatives to antibiotics that may be gentler on the digestive system.

Chapter 9:

Two-Week Meal Plan

Take care of your body. It is the only place you have to live. –Jim Rohn

We've almost reached the end of this journey in learning more about gut health, but now we've reached the point where you take the reins and begin your path to better health. This is not the time when I'll ask you to throw away all the junk food that you have in your pantry. This journey is yours, and you need to do what feels right for you. Instead, I'll ask you to simply add some basic staple items to your fridge and pantry so that you have healthy ingredients on hand when it's time to cook. The idea is to get curious about new foods and recipes so that you can explore what will best serve your body and mind. I want to help you get started on this path by providing you with some of the meal plans and recipes that have helped me on my personal journey. If, in your quest to make healthier meals, you feel like you'll be short-changing yourself of exotic flavors or engaging meals, think again, because these recipes will leave you satisfied with the bonus of not making you feel sick or sluggish. Feel free to adapt, supplement, replace, add, or even ignore certain foods within these recipes to best suit your needs and tastes. Remember that this is for you, so make healthy revisions as needed so that mealtime is exciting and fun.

Meal Plans

The following meal plans and recipes are primarily plant-based, gluten-free, and vegan. For many people, if they limit or eliminate the amount of meat, gluten, and dairy in their diet, they notice an improvement in digestion, so these recipes center around that idea. Since these plans are simply a guide for meal ideas, feel free to add animal proteins like salmon, chicken, or other options to make the meals practical for your needs. It's never too early or too late to start working toward better health, so get planning!

Week 1:

	Monday	Tuesday	Wednesday	Thursday	Friday	Saturday	Sunday
Breakfast	Gluten-free Blueberry Muffins	Mint Chip Smoothie	Chia seeds and Strawberry Pudding	Basil Mango Smoothie	Quinoa Cinnamon Porridge	Green Goddess Smoothie	Mint Chip Smoothie
Lunch	Buddha Bowl	Mushroom Lettuce Cups	Greek Salad	Herb Flatbread with Tomato Soup	Zoodles with Hemp Seed Pesto	Gluten-free Pasta with Veggies	Greek Salad
Dinner	Gluten-free Pad Thai	Quinoa and Kale Salad	Buddha Bowl	Mushroom Lettuce Cups	Herb Flatbread with Tomato Soup	Zoodles and Hemp Seed Pesto	Zoodles with Hemp Seed Pesto

Week 2:

	Monday	Tuesday	Wednesday	Thursday	Friday	Saturday	Sunday
Breakfast	Avocado Toast	Green Goddess Smoothie	Fruit and Coconut Yogurt Bowl	Basil and Mango Smoothie	Quinoa Cinnamon Porridge	Chocolate Chia Seed Pudding	Fruit and Coconut Yogurt Bowl
Lunch	Taco Salad	Black Bean Soup	Buddha Bowl	Gluten-free Vegan Mac and Cheese	Butternut Squash Soup	Gluten-free Pad Thai	Spring Rolls with Peanut Sauce
Dinner	Quinoa and Kale Salad	Gluten-free Vegan Mac and Cheese	Butternut Squash Soup	Taco Salad Spring Rolls with Peanut Sauce	Buddha Bowl	Taco Salad	Black Bean Soup

Recipes for Optimal Gut Health

Breakfast Options:

Avocado Toast

This recipe is one of my all-time favorites and, while I've placed it in the breakfast category, I find myself eating it for breakfast, lunch, or dinner. The avocado and lemon give a great balance of flavors, and I feel energized every time I eat this. Enjoy!

Total Time: 5 minutes

Serving Size: 1–2

Prep Time: 5 minutes

Ingredients:

- 2 pieces of sourdough* or gluten-free bread (toasted)
- 1 avocado
- 1 tbsp olive oil
- 1 tbsp fresh lemon juice
- 1/2 tsp black pepper
- 1/2 tsp garlic powder
- 1 tsp sea salt
- Optional: hot sauce, red pepper flakes (to taste)

*Sourdough bread contains gluten, but the fermentation process helps the body break down gluten for easier digestion.

Directions:

1. In a medium bowl, mash the avocado.

2. Add the olive oil, lemon juice, black pepper, garlic powder, sea salt, and hot sauce/red pepper flakes (if desired).

3. Spread the mixture on the toasted bread. Add a bit of olive oil and sea salt on top if desired.

Gluten-Free Blueberry Muffins

If you crave those baked goods but know the ones you buy in the bakery section can make you feel sluggish, try these gluten-free blueberry muffins instead. These are made with simple and delicious ingredients that leave your sweet tooth satisfied with the subtly-sweet flavors of honey, vanilla, and blueberries.

Total Time: 30 minutes

Serving Size: 12 muffins

Prep Time: 10 minutes

Cook Time: 20 minutes

Ingredients:

- 2 cups gluten-free or almond baking flour
- 1/2 tsp baking soda
- 1/2 tsp sea salt

- 3 eggs

- 3 tbsp monk fruit sweetener

- 1 tsp vanilla extract

- 2 tbsp coconut oil

- 3 tbsp ghee or butter (grass-fed) or butter substitute

- 2 tbsp honey

- 1 cup fresh blueberries

Directions:

1. Heat oven to 350 degrees.

2. In a large bowl, combine the dry ingredients thoroughly.

3. Add all the wet ingredients and stir well.

4. Once ingredients are well combined, add in the blueberries and gently mix.

5. Line muffin pans or grease with coconut oil and fill tins 3/4 of the way.

6. Bake at 350 for 20 minutes or until muffins are golden on the top.

Basil and Mango Smoothie

Smoothies are a great way to jumpstart any day, and this one is packed with healthy foods that will keep you satisfied for several hours. The half-cup of spinach adds more vitamins to this smoothie, while the blended drink will still taste like a sweet blend of fruits.

Total Time: 10 minutes

Serving Size: 1

Prep Time: 10 minutes

Ingredients:

- 1 frozen banana
- 1 1/2 cups basil
- 1 cup fresh or frozen mango
- 1 1/2 cups packed spinach
- Optional: 1 tsp spirulina
- Optional: sweeteners such as honey

Directions:

1. Mix ingredients in a blender for 2–3 minutes. Add sweeteners like sugar, Stevia, or honey if desired.
2. Pour into your favorite glass or travel cup and enjoy!

Green Goddess Smoothie

This smoothie is designed to ramp up your day from the first sip (no coffee needed!). The avocado gives the dish a smooth texture, while the coconut milk adds a creaminess. You'll definitely feel the energy after drinking this one.

Total Time: 10 minutes

Serving Size: 1

Prep Time: 10 minutes

Ingredients:

- 1 cup kale

- 2 cups spinach

- 1/2 an avocado

- 1/2 cup frozen or fresh mango

- 12 oz coconut milk

- 1/3 cup ice cubes

- 1 tbsp hemp seeds

- 1 tbsp chia seeds

- Optional: sweeteners such as honey

Directions:

1. Mix every ingredient together in a blender for 2–3 minutes. Add sweeteners like sugar, Stevia, or honey if desired.

2. Pour into your favorite glass or travel cup and enjoy!

Fruit and Coconut Yogurt Bowl

For a wholesome start to the day, this fruit and yogurt combination will taste delicious and give you a sweet treat. The more varieties of fruits you have in this bowl, the better, so pick your favorites and change them up often.

Total Time: 3–5 minutes

Serving Size: 1

Prep Time: 3–5 minutes

Ingredients:

- 1/2 cup of your choice of fruit (strawberries, blueberries, kiwi, mango, pineapple, pomegranate seeds, banana, etc.)

- 1/2 cup coconut milk yogurt

- Optional: sweetener such as maple syrup, cocoa powder, or honey

Directions:

1. Use a medium bowl to stir the coconut milk yogurt and fruit together.

2. Add a drizzle of sweetener if preferred (honey, cocoa powder, cacao nibs, maple syrup).

Chia Seed and Strawberry Pudding

The crunchy, naturally sweet ingredients of this recipe can act as an alternative to sugary cakes or puddings. This treat will leave you feeling refreshed and keep your stomach feeling happy.

Total Time: 8+ hours (fridge time included)

Serving Size: 1

Prep Time: 10 minutes

Fridge Time: 6–8 hours to set (or overnight)

Ingredients:

- 1 1/2 cups strawberries

- 4 tbsp chia seeds

- 1 cup of coconut milk

- Optional: add any additional fruits you love

- Optional: sweeteners such as honey or maple syrup

- Optional: additional toppings (chopped strawberries, coconut flakes, cocoa powder)

Directions:

1. Blend the strawberries and coconut milk to your desired texture (pureed smooth or a bit chunky).

2. Add any additional fruit (if desired) and blend for 30 more seconds.

3. Add the chia seeds and any sweeteners that you want (honey, maple syrup, Stevia, etc.) and stir.

4. Leave the mixture in the fridge overnight, or for 6–8 hours at least.

5. Once refrigerated fully, add additional toppings if desired and enjoy!

Chocolate Chia Seed Pudding

I used to love ice cream, but it never loved me. This recipe satisfies my love of that sweet, cold, chocolatey taste without giving my stomach any trouble later. This is a perfect one for a hot, summer day.

Total Time: 8+ hours (fridge time included)

Serving Size: 1

Prep Time: 10 minutes

Fridge Time: 6–8 hours to set (or overnight)

Ingredients:

- 4 tbsp chia seeds

- 2 tbsp maple syrup

- 4 tbsp cacao powder

- 1 cup coconut milk

- Optional: bananas, coconut flakes for topping

Directions:

1. Blend the maple syrup, cacao powder, and coconut milk to your desired texture (pureed smooth or a bit chunky).

2. Add the chia seeds and blend for 30 more seconds.

3. Leave the mixture in the fridge overnight, or for 6–8 hours at least.

4. Once refrigerated fully, add additional toppings like bananas or coconut flakes if desired, and enjoy!

Lunch and Dinner Options:

Gluten-Free/Vegan Mac 'n' Cheese

If you crave a satisfying, creamy meal, this one's for you. The 'cheese' sauce created to pair with the pasta gives a wholesome, hearty meal, and the spinach adds extra nutrients and protein.

Total Time: 15–20 minutes

Serving Size: 3–4

Prep Time: 10–15 minutes

Cook Time: 5–6 minutes

Ingredients:

- 2 cups spinach
- 1 pkg gluten-free pasta

Sauce:

- 5 tbsp nutritional yeast
- 4 garlic cloves
- 3 tbsp avocado oil
- 1/2 cup cashews (soaked in water for 2–4 hours before boiling)
- 1/2 tsp black pepper
- 1/2 sea salt
- 1 cup water

Directions:

1. Follow directions on the package to cook the pasta.
2. Combine cheese sauce ingredients in a blender and puree until smooth.
3. In a pan, heat the cheese sauce on the stovetop for a minute.
4. Mix spinach into the cheese sauce and cook for 3–4 minutes.

5. Mix cooked pasta into the cheese until combined and heated.

Zoodles with Hemp Seed Pesto

This is a great fall or winter meal that is quick and easy when you don't have much time. The lemon juice and olives add a lot of flavors to this meal, so make sure to include these ingredients.

Total Time: 10–15 minutes

Serving Size: 2–3

Prep Time: 10–15 minutes

Ingredients:

- 2 zucchinis

- 1/2 cup cherry tomatoes (halved)

- 1/4 cup kalamata olives

- **Pesto Sauce:**

- 1 lemon (juiced)

- 2 cups fresh basil

- 3/4 cup of hemp seeds

- 1/2 cup olive oil

- 4–5 garlic cloves

- 1 tsp black pepper

- 1 tsp sea salt

Directions:

1. Use a spiralizer or shredder to spiral the zucchini in a large bowl to make 'zoodles.'

2. Blend or food process the pesto ingredients together until well combined.

3. Cover the 'zoodles' with the sauce and add the tomatoes and olives.

Gluten-Free Pasta with Veggies

If you miss pasta because you gave it up after it impacted your digestive system, get excited about this next recipe. Most mainstream grocery stores carry gluten-free pasta that can be used as a substitute for the real thing. The variety of veggies in this recipe gives even more taste and texture to this dish. You'll want a second helping after trying this one.

Total Time: 20–30 minutes

Serving Size: 2–4

Prep Time: 15–20 minutes

Cook Time: 10 minutes (pasta)

Ingredients:

- 6 oz cooked gluten-free pasta of your choice

- 1 large carrot (chopped into rounds)

- 1/2 red onion (chopped)

- 1 radish (sliced and cut into fourths)

- 1/2 yellow bell pepper (chopped)

- 1 cup cilantro (roughly chopped)

- 1 jalapeño (sliced)

Dressing:

- 1/2 lemon (juiced)

- 4 garlic cloves (minced)

- 2 tsp apple cider vinegar

- 3 tbsp olive oil

- 1/2 tsp red pepper flakes

- 1/2 tsp black pepper

- 1/2 tsp sea salt

Directions:

1. Follow directions to cook pasta.

2. In a large bowl, combine all the vegetables.

3. Add cooked pasta to the vegetable mixture.

4. In a small bowl, combine all the dressing ingredients.

5. Mix the dressing into the mixed vegetables and pasta until thoroughly combined.

Mushroom Lettuce Cups

I've learned to love mushrooms since they take on the taste of the flavors around them. The leaf lettuce used in this recipe gives a healthy alternative to buns and bread. The combination of flavors is bold and satisfying.

Total Time: 15–20 minutes

Serving Size: 3–4

Prep Time: 5 minutes

Cook Time: 10–12 minutes

Ingredients:

- 12 butter leaf lettuce cups
- 3/4 cup green onions
- 6 cups white mushrooms
- 1 tbsp ginger
- 3 tbsp tamari
- 2 tbsp sesame oil
- 3 garlic cloves
- 1/2 tsp black pepper
- 1 tbsp white wine vinegar
- 3 tbsp sriracha

Directions:

1. In a pan, heat the sesame oil over medium heat. Add the mushrooms and cook, stirring often, for 3–5 minutes.

2. Stir in garlic, green onions, ginger, black pepper, white wine vinegar, and sriracha. Let this mixture cook for 7 minutes. Mushrooms should be cooked through.

3. Scoop mixture into lettuce cups and serve.

Buddha Bowl

This filling recipe is great when you have guests that love gut health as much as you do. The ingredients create a healthy meal but also allow you to feel satisfied with the hearty ingredients like quinoa and sweet potatoes.

Total Time: 30 minutes

Serving Size: 2–4

Prep Time: 10–15 minutes

Cook Time: 20–25 minutes

Ingredients:

- 1 cup quinoa (cooked)
- 1/2 avocado (sliced)
- 1 cup cremini or white mushrooms (sliced)
- 1/2 cup arugula
- 1 sweet potato (cubed)
- 1 cup snap peas
- 1 tbsp grass-fed butter or butter substitute

Pesto Sauce:

- 1 lemon (juiced)
- 3/4 cup of hemp seeds
- 2 cups of basil (fresh)

- 4–5 garlic cloves

- 1/2 cup olive oil

- 1 tsp black pepper

- 1 tsp sea salt

Directions:

1. Preheat oven to 375 degrees.

2. Once chopped, place sweet potatoes on a baking sheet. Pour a drizzle of olive oil and combine. Sprinkle salt and pepper over the potatoes. Bake for 20 minutes.

3. While potatoes cook, melt butter or butter substitute over medium heat. Add the snap peas and mushrooms and cook, stirring often, for 10 minutes.

4. Blend the pesto ingredients in a blender or food processor until smooth.

5. Place cooked quinoa in a bowl and add the vegetables, sweet potatoes, and arugula.

6. Add pesto and avocado to the top.

Greek Salad

For a lighter meal that definitely delivers on taste, try this one for lunch or dinner. The blend of spices in the dressing is tasty and flavorful.

Total Time: 10–15 minutes

Serving Size: 2–4

Prep Time: 10–15 minutes

Ingredients:

Salad:

- 3 cups romaine lettuce (chopped)
- 1/2 cup chopped red onion
- 1/2 cup cherry tomatoes (halved)
- 1/2 cup chopped cucumber
- 1/2 cup pepperoncini
- 1/4 cup kalamata olives (halved)
- 1/4 cup red pepper (sliced)

Dressing:

- 1/2 lemon (juiced)
- 2 tbsp olive oil
- 1/2 tsp oregano flakes
- 1/4 tsp black pepper
- 1/4 tsp sea salt
- 2 tsp white wine vinegar
- 2 garlic cloves (minced)

Directions:

1. Combine all the dressing ingredients in a small bowl.
2. Combine salad ingredients together in a medium bowl.
3. Pour dressing over salad and stir well (until coated evenly).

Tomato Soup and Herb Flatbread

On a cold day, what's better than tomato soup? This recipe maximizes the boldness of the flavors in the soup. Soak it all up with the homemade flatbread and enjoy!

Total Time: 30 minutes

Serving Size: 1–2

Prep Time: 5–10 minutes

Cook Time: 20 minutes

Ingredients:

Soup:

- 2 tbsp grass-fed butter or butter substitute
- 2 tbsp olive oil
- 1 medium onion
- 3 garlic cloves
- 3 tbsp tomato paste
- 1 tsp sea salt
- 1/4 cup basil
- 2 cups vegetable stock
- 1 can whole tomatoes with juice
- black pepper (to taste)

Flatbread:

- 1 1/2 cup almond flour

- 1 tbsp chia seeds

- 3 garlic cloves

- 1 tbsp chopped rosemary

- 1/4 tsp sea salt

- 2 tbsp grass-fed butter or butter substitute

- 1 tsp apple cider vinegar

Directions:

Soup:

1. Heat butter and oil over medium heat in a saucepan. Add the onion and sea salt. Cook (covered) for 10 minutes, stirring often.

2. Add canned tomatoes and their juice to the pan.

3. Add vegetable stock. Bring the mixture to a boil, reduce the heat, and simmer for 20 minutes.

4. Blend the soup until smooth and add sea salt and black pepper.

Flatbread:

1. Preheat oven to 375 degrees. Put chia seeds in a small bowl of warm water for 10 minutes to thicken.

2. Mix all the ingredients except chia seeds and vinegar.

3. Once every ingredient is stirred well, add the chia seeds and apple cider vinegar.

4. Roll mixture into two flatbreads and bake for 10 minutes.

Butternut Squash Soup

This is another homemade classic that will taste creamy and delicious. It's a delightful dish for guests or to make just for yourself and store in the fridge or freezer to reheat later.

Total Time: 50 minutes

Serving Size: 3–4

Prep Time: 10 minutes

Cook Time: 40 minutes

Ingredients:

- 1 yellow onion (chopped)

- 2 sweet potatoes (cubed)

- 2 carrots (chopped into rounds)

- 2 stalks celery (chopped)

- 1 butternut squash (peeled, seeded, and cubed)

- 2 tbsp grass-fed butter or butter substitute

- 32 oz vegetable stock

- 1 1/2 tsp sea salt

- 2 tsp black pepper

- 2 tsp garlic powder

Directions:

1. Heat butter over medium heat in a large pot. Add the celery, onions, carrots, sweet potatoes, and squash. Cook for 5 minutes, stirring often, until the vegetables are tender.

2. Mix in the garlic powder, vegetable stock, black pepper, and sea salt.

3. Bring to a boil, cover pot, and reduce heat to low. Simmer for 35 minutes.

4. Allow to cool, then puree the soup in a blender until smooth.

Black Bean Soup

This soup is great for a cold winter day and is packed with protein that will keep you feeling alert. The chipotle chili powder gives it a nice kick and can be adjusted according to taste.

Total Time: 30 minutes

Serving Size: 3–4

Prep Time: 5 minutes

Cook Time: 25 minutes

Ingredients:

- 2 cans of black beans (drained and rinsed)

- 4 cups of vegetable stock or broth

- 1 large onion (sliced)

- 4 garlic cloves (minced)

- 1 bunch of cilantros (roughly chopped)

- 3 tbsp olive oil

- 1 1/2 tsp sea salt

- 1 tsp chili powder

- 1 1/2 tsp cumin

- 1/2 tsp chipotle chili powder

- 1 tsp black pepper

- Optional: fresh lime, avocado, gluten-free tortilla chips

Directions:

1. Use a large pot to heat the olive oil over medium heat. Mix in the sliced onion and salt. Cook for 5 minutes, stirring often.

2. Mix the garlic and spices into the pot with the onion. Cover and cook for 5 minutes.

3. Mix the beans, vegetable stock or broth, and cilantro into the pot. Bring this to a boil and let it simmer for 15 minutes.

4. Allow the mixture to cool and blend the soup in a blender until smooth.

Taco Salad

Tacos have always been one of my favorite meals because of the variety of ingredients that can be included. This taco salad is a healthy variation of the taco, but it doesn't hold back on flavor. The dressing for this salad is delicious with the blended flavors of jalapeños, avocado, and garlic.

Total Time: 10–15 minutes

Serving Size: 2–4

Prep Time: 5–10 minutes

Ingredients:

Dressing:

- 1 jalapeño
- 3 garlic cloves
- 1/2 avocado
- 3 tbsp water
- 1 tbsp olive oil
- 2 limes (juiced)
- 1/2 tsp black pepper
- 1/2 tsp sea salt

Salad:

- 2 cups arugula
- 3 cups romaine lettuce
- 1/2 cup red onion (diced)
- 1/2 cup cherry tomatoes (halved)
- 1/2 avocado (sliced)
- 1 cup cilantro leaves (roughly chopped)

Directions:

1. Place all the ingredients for the dressing in a blender or food processor and blend/puree until smooth.

2. Combine salad ingredients and drizzle the dressing over top. Serve!

Gluten-Free Pad Thai

This healthy, wholesome spin on regular pad Thai is quick, filling, and makes the perfect dish to share with others. It's full of delicious, crunchy veggies that give the meal texture and flavor. I love the combination of peanut butter and ginger for the sauce.

Total Time: 15 minutes

Serving Size: 2–4

Prep Time: 5 minutes

Cook Time: 10 minutes

Ingredients:

- 6 oz gluten-free fettuccine noodles (cooked)
- 1 orange bell pepper (sliced)
- 1 red bell pepper (sliced)
- 2 jalapeños (sliced)
- 1 cup bean sprouts
- 1 cup cilantro leaves
- 1/2 cup chopped green onions

- 2 tbsp avocado oil

Sauce:

- 1 piece of ginger (peeled)

- 3 garlic cloves

- 1/4 cup plus 1 tbsp of peanut butter

- 3 tbsp tamari

- 1/4 and 1 tbsp water

- 1/2 tsp black pepper

- 1/2 tsp sea salt

- 1 tbsp sriracha

Directions:

1. In a deep pan or wok, heat the avocado oil over medium heat.

2. Stir in bell peppers and cook for 3–4 minutes.

3. While peppers cook, place all the sauce ingredients into a blender and puree until smooth.

4. Add the bean sprouts, jalapeños, and green onions to the bell peppers. Stir and cook for 2 minutes.

5. Mix the sauce and cooked noodles in the pan with the vegetables until warmed through and thoroughly combined (1–2 minutes).

Spring Rolls with Peanut Sauce

If you love the Pad Thai recipe, you'll love the flavors in this one as well. It packs in the microgreens and veggies while pairing well with the spicy-sweet sauce.

Total Time: 15–20 minutes

Serving Size: 3–4

Prep Time: 10 minutes

Ingredients:

- 1 1/2 cups bean sprouts or other microgreens
- 8 sheets of rice paper or spring roll paper
- 1 1/2 cups carrots (julienned)
- 1 1/2 cups spinach (roughly chopped)
- 1 cup fresh mint
- 1 1/2 cups red cabbage (sliced)
- 1 cup cilantro (chopped)

Sauce:

- 1/2 cup peanut butter
- 1/4 cup rice vinegar
- 1/2 tbsp ginger (grated)
- 1/4 cup tamari
- 1/4 cup water
- 3 garlic cloves

- 1 tbsp sriracha

- 2 tbsp avocado oil

Directions:

1. Fill a bowl with lukewarm water. Dip a sheet of rice paper in the water until it is wet and softened. Move rice paper to a cutting board or flat, clean surface.

2. Add some spinach, red cabbage, mint, cilantro, bean sprouts, and some carrots to one side of the paper. Starting with the vegetable side, roll the paper like a burrito (tuck in the vegetables). Continue doing this for the remaining wraps.

3. Puree all the sauce ingredients in a blender until smooth.

4. Serve the rolls with peanut sauce.

Kale and Quinoa Salad

If you've never tried kale and quinoa before, this combination is both satisfying and tasty. The red pepper flakes add some spicy flavoring to this salad, and the mixture of spices adds bold, new flavors.

Total Time: 10 minutes

Serving Size: 2–3

Prep Time: 10 minutes

Ingredients:

- 1/2 cup cooked quinoa

- 1 bunch dino' kale

- 4 garlic cloves (minced)

- 3 tbsp olive oil

- 1 lemon (juiced)

- 2 tsp red pepper flakes

- 1 tsp black pepper

- 1 tsp sea salt

Directions:

1. Chop kale leaves into thin strips, removing the ribs.

2. Mix kale leaves and lemon juice in a large bowl. Mix in a small drizzle of olive oil.

3. In a medium bowl, combine lemon juice, garlic, olive oil, sea salt, black pepper, and red pepper flakes and mix together.

4. Mix the quinoa, kale, and dressing together in a large bowl until combined. Enjoy!

Bon Appetit

I've always been a food lover but didn't know how to balance my love of flavors with my desire to keep my stomach happy and healthy until I got wiser about my gut health. In researching what foods and spices would keep my digestive tract performing at its best, I made discoveries in new pairings of foods, and I continue to explore this when I cook. I find that I now have more use for my spice rack than I ever did before when adding flavors to the vegetables in my meals.

While these veggies are delicious on their own, I've learned ways to create new combinations that I love. This makes cooking, new and exciting for me each time I prepare a meal.

If you haven't cooked much for yourself in the past, open your mind to this new opportunity. Get experimental with interesting flavors and spices. In this case, the more new spices you can experiment with, the better. Try to include as many colorful vegetables as possible in your meals. These can brighten up dishes that you might have found boring in the past. One of the best parts of cooking meals is that you get to control what ingredients are added to the dishes, so you know what healthy whole foods are going into your meals. Get creative, try new foods, and share your dishes with others. Happy cooking!

Conclusion

Your body holds deep wisdom. Trust in it. Learn from it. Nourish it. Watch your life transform and be healthy. –Bella Bleue

When our bodies feel good, we tend to be better versions of ourselves. We are more willing to go on new adventures, live life to the fullest, and share our happiness with others. When feeling healthy is an option for people, it's amazing to see how many choose not to take advantage of this gift. Many choose the easy, available, quick solution that will keep them feeling hungry and dissatisfied. Together, we can change this thinking. Continue to educate yourself about gut health and use this journey as a reminder of what goals you'd like to accomplish. You've come a long way, and you should feel proud of yourself. Even if you're still in the planning stages of finding time to eat healthier, exercise, and take better care of your mind, you've learned promising strategies that will help you make lifestyle changes so that you can feel better. By committing to continuing this journey, you are making a pledge to reward yourself with a stronger sense of self and a feeling of rejuvenation.

Good gut health needs to be something you are comfortable practicing consistently and easily. Otherwise, it becomes a chore. This means that eating, exercise, and self-care efforts need to feel routine, so they flow into your schedule even when you're busy and tired. Choose practices that will be healthy for you and ones that you will be able to continue to maintain because you like doing them. When you include these things that make your body feel good, your body will reward you with the ability to be more active and energized as you go about your day. This is one of the best outcomes of good gut health and, once you put some preparation into learning about diverse foods, exercises, and self-care habits that you like, you'll be able to enjoy how your body and mind feel.

Remind yourself often that the role of the gut should be to take the best, healthiest vitamins and minerals from the foods and liquids you consume and turn them into fuel for your body. When this happens successfully, tissue is repaired, nutrients are properly absorbed, and energy is produced. It doesn't take an entire upheaval in one's life to start making simple dietary changes for the better. It simply requires a start to this progress.

By following the six steps outlined throughout the chapters, you'll be well on your way to living a calmer, healthier life. We give ourselves power when we learn to cut out certain foods, reset our systems, heal the gut, maintain a routine, move our bodies, and practice self-care. Creating daily habits for good gut health will make any changes you've made to your life easier to implement. Others may not see this journey as you do because they may not have the insight and knowledge you now possess. Remember that you are only in control of the choices that you make and the things you decide to eat. By staying positive on this journey, you will set a tone for others to stand in awe of and possibly gravitate toward.

The two-week meal plan and recipes that you now have access to in this book will give you an easy start with changing your habits so that you don't need to overthink the things you can eat. The whole foods used in these recipes will provide you with healthier options that will satisfy your cravings and leave you feeling natural energy in your body and mind. Knowing that digestion is so closely linked with mental health gives us a fighting chance to focus more on the way we care for our minds and include self-care practices specifically designed to calm anxiety so that gut health improves. Let this journey move you to make deeper realizations about yourself, your body, and your mind, then adjust as you continue your quest for good gut health.

Make a Commitment to Yourself

When I was on that plane so long ago, experiencing my first panic attack, I never thought it would lead me on this rocky journey to rethink the way I consider eating or living, but here I am. My advice to you is to continue the conversation on gut health in your own social circles because you'll probably discover others with commonalities that could benefit. I have found my own wide circle of friends who have struggled with digestive issues in the past and now continue to be mindful every day when eating and caring for themselves. This group has made me feel powerful and confident that remaining quiet about gut health will be a thing of the past. This topic needs a spotlight shining brightly on it, so don't be afraid to speak out on the importance of this issue.

By changing the way we treat the digestive system, we make a choice to value this vital issue. With a commitment to caring for our gut, we show our body that we think it's important enough to want to live in it a little longer and with purpose. Imagine your life with a functioning digestive system that doesn't slow you down or take time away from activities that you love. This life is a possibility when you seriously consider what needs to change and when you start making intentional choices for yourself. One of the best decisions you can make is to educate yourself on your body and the ways that it can perform at its finest for you. The introduction of fast, fried, processed foods into our society was an unfortunate setback for many in terms of gut health, and we still have a long way to go in making these realizations known to the public. It doesn't need to be too late to make changes for yourself and your life, though. By making conscious choices to include more whole foods in your diet each day, you fill your body with the nourishment that will sustain you so that you can avoid junk foods. Make a commitment for your digestive health but also for your life. Experience this new way of living for yourself and appreciate the work that you've done to get here, then share this life with others.

Glossary

Ashwagandha Mushroom: A type of mushroom said to promote sleep help and relaxation by relaxing the body and mind.

Bitters: A type of herb, root, or plant that has been soaked in aromatics like peppermint or lemongrass to bring out its complex flavors and properties.

Collagen: A protein found in the body that works to hold cells together. A collagen supplement can work to hold cells together as aging occurs.

Diaphragmatic Breathing: Designed to calm stress, this is a system of breathing where a person focuses on the air moving into and out of the abdomen as they slowly breathe.

Dopamine: A neurotransmitter of the brain that acts as an assistant in body functions, memory, and mood.

Enteric Nervous System (ENS): A layer of nerve cells that controls digestion and assists with the absorption of nutrients in the body.

Gut Health: The health of the digestive system in its entirety, from the esophagus to the bowel. This focus influences the health and well-being of an individual's body and mental state.

Immune Function: The making and activity of cells that prevent illness.

Lavender: A plant with a pleasant smell that provides natural stress and pain relief.

Leaky Gut Syndrome: The idea that permeability forms in the intestines as a symptom of gastrointestinal disease, leading to toxins released into the bloodstream.

Lemon Balm: An herb containing chemicals that promote relaxation and help in the reduction of illnesses.

Licorice Root: Sold as a supplement, this root is thought to promote digestive health by relieving inflammation.

L-glutamine: An acid that heals the intestinal lining and can help prevent digestive conditions.

Marshmallow Root: An herb thought to aid in healing and digestive health by flushing out toxins in the body.

Microbiome: The microorganisms, such as bacteria, that make up certain areas of the human body.

Neuroinflammation: The response within the brain or spine that causes inflammation when gut health is neglected.

Neurotransmitters: Chemical transmitters within the body that move messages or signals from one part of the body to another.

Prebiotics: A food source for the body's healthy bacteria so that this bacteria can benefit the digestive tract.

Probiotics: Good bacteria living in the body, including live yeast. This kind of good bacteria keeps the body feeling healthy and balanced.

Reishi Mushroom: A mushroom that is said to strengthen the immune system and fight illness.

Rhodiola Rosea: A root that is said to decrease anxiety by assisting in stress and fatigue reduction.

Serotonin: A chemical that plays a major role in overall health and performance because it moves messages from the brain to other parts of the body. It is vital for controlling mood, bone health, and sleep.

The Vagus Nerve: The nerve that travels from the brain to the body and controls aspects of digestion and the immune system.

Whole Foods: Foods that are in their original form and minimally processed or not processed in order to gain the most nutritional value from the food.

Helpful Apps and Resources

for Gut Health

Down Dog: This app is a simple and helpful one for incorporating yoga and meditation into your day. https://downdogapp.com/

Viome: This website is an at-home gut health test to give a person information about foods and supplements that will best benefit them. https://viome.com/

Yuka: This app is a product scanner for food and beauty products. This will inform a customer about information and ingredients in a product and will provide a health grade for that product. https://apps.apple.com/us/app/yuka-food-cosmetic-scanner/id1092799236

Leave a Quick Amazon Review!

References

A quote by Karyn Calabrese. (n.d.). Goodreads. Retrieved August 25, 2022, from https://goodreads.com/quotes/381031-if-you-don-t-take-care-of-this-the-most-magnificent

Anderer, J. (2021, July 14). *New Study Reveals a Huge Side Effect of Walking More.* Eat This Not That. https://eatthis.com/news-does-walking-improve-memory/#:~:text=%22Walking%20encourages%20our%20brain%20to

Are omega-6 fatty acids linked to heart disease? (2021, December 17). Mayo Clinic. https://mayoclinic.org/diseases-conditions/heart-disease/expert-answers/omega-6/faq-20058172

Balance in the body is the foundation for balance in life. - B.K.S. Iyengar quotes. (n.d.). Statustown. Retrieved August 23, 2022, from https://statustown.com/quote/896/#:~:text=Balance%20in%20the%20body%20is

Being Healthy Starts in Your Gut: Tips for Promoting Optimal Gut Health and Preventing Disease. (2017, June 18). Sunrise Hospital and Medical Center. https://sunrisehospital.com/about/newsroom/being-healthy-starts-in-your-gut-tips-for-promoting-optimal-gut-health-and-preventing-disease

Bhattacharya, S. (2020). *The Role of Spirulina (Arthrospira) in the Mitigation of Heavy-Metal Toxicity: An Appraisal.* Journal of Environmental Pathology, Toxicology and Oncology, 39(2), 149–157.

https://doi.org/10.1615/jenvironpatholtoxicoloncol.20
20034375

Blasi, E. (2021, September 23). *Working Out According to Your Menstrual Cycle Stages*. Oxygen Mag. https://oxygenmag.com/training-tips-for-women/working-out-according-to-your-menstrual-cycle-stages/

Boghos, R. (2020, January 14). *Detox Naturally With Tongue Scraping*. Energy Matters LLC - Rose Boghos. https://energymattersllc.com/blogs/news/detox-naturally-with-tongue-scraping

Braun, A., & Caplan, E. (2021, July 28). *These 10 Herbal Teas Can Help You Reduce Your Stress and Improve Your Brain Health*. Healthline. https://healthline.com/health/mental-health/tea-for-stress

Breus, D. M. (2022, June 27). *The Relationship Between Sleep and Stress*. The Sleep Doctor. https://thesleepdoctor.com/mental-health/stress-and-sleep/

Brown, M. J. (2019, October 22). *What Are Advanced Glycation End Products (AGEs)?* Healthline; Healthline Media. https://healthline.com/nutrition/advanced-glycation-end-products

Cajigal, S. (2021, October). *Exploring the Link Between Gut and Brain Health*. brainandlife.org. https://brainandlife.org/articles/exploring-link-between-gut-brain-health/

CDC Newsroom. (2016, January 1). CDC. https://cdc.gov/media/releases/2016/p0215-enough-

sleep.html#:~:text=The%20American%20Academy%2
0of%20Sleep

Charbel, H. (2018, February 23). *10 Ways to Keep Your Microbiome Healthy - Dr. Halim Charbel, Maryland.* Digestive Care Specialists. https://digestivecare-specialists.com/10-ways-to-keep-your-microbiome-healthy/

Chen, L., Zhu, Y., Hu, Z., Wu, S., & Jin, C. (2021). *Beetroot as a functional food with huge health benefits: Antioxidant, antitumor, physical function, and chronic metabolomics activity.* Food Science & Nutrition, 9(11), 6406–6420. https://doi.org/10.1002/fsn3.2577

Clauss, M., Gerard, P., Mosca, A., & Leclerc, M. (2021, June 10). *Interplay Between Exercise and Gut Microbiome in the Context of Human Health and Performance.* Frontiers in Nutrition.
https://frontiersin.org/articles/10.3389/fnut.2021.637
010/full#:~:text=Moderate%20exercise%20has%20po
sitive%20effects,produced%20in%20the%20gastrointes
tinal%20tract

Cleveland Clinic. (2020, March 9). *Probiotics: What is it, benefits, side effects, food & types.* Cleveland Clinic. https://my.clevelandclinic.org/health/articles/14598-probiotics

Cleveland Clinic. (2022a, March 14). *Neurotransmitters: What They Are, Functions & Types.* Cleveland Clinic. https://my.clevelandclinic.org/health/articles/22513-neurotransmitters#:~:text=What%20are%20neurotrans
mitters%3F

Cleveland Clinic. (2022b, March 18). *Serotonin: What Is It, Function & Levels.* Cleveland Clinic. https://my.clevelandclinic.org/health/articles/22572-

serotonin#:~:text=Serotonin%20is%20a%20chemical
%20that

Cleveland Clinic. (2022c, March 23). *Dopamine: What It Is, Function & Symptoms.* Cleveland Clinic. https://my.clevelandclinic.org/health/articles/22581-dopamine#:~:text=Dopamine%20is%20a%20neurotra nsmitter%20made

Clifford, E. (2021, October 15). *How to Reset Your Body After Eating Unhealthy.* Erin Clifford Wellness Coaching. https://erincliffordwellness.com/resetting-body-after-eating-unhealthy/#:~:text=Drink%20herbal%20tea%20instea d%20to

Collins, J. (2020, September 14). *What Are Prebiotics?* WebMD. https://webmd.com/digestive-disorders/prebiotics-overview

Coyle, D. (2017, June 19). *8 Surprising Things That Harm Your Gut Bacteria.* Healthline. https://healthline.com/nutrition/8-things-that-harm-gut-bacteria#TOC_TITLE_HDR_2

Cronkleton, E. (2017, September 21). *Marshmallow Root: Benefits, Side Effects, and More.* Healthline. https://healthline.com/health/food-nutrition/marshmallow-root#digestion

Dehbi, A. (2019, February 15). *Immediate Benefits of Improved Gut Health.* Prime (Keepmeprime.com). https://keepmeprime.com/benefits-improved-gut-health-immediate/

Differences in Organic, Natural, and Health Foods. (2021, August 6). HealthyChildren.org. https://healthychildren.org/English/healthy-living/nutrition/Pages/Differences-in-Organic-Natural-and-Health-Foods.aspx#:~:text=Organic%20foods%20are%20grown%20without

DiSabato, D. J., Quan, N., & Godbout, J. P. (2016). *Neuroinflammation: the devil is in the details.* Journal of Neurochemistry, 139, 136–153. https://doi.org/10.1111/jnc.13607

Do you have a hormonal imbalance? (2022, March 4). Geisinger.org. https://geisinger.org/health-and-wellness/wellness-articles/2022/03/04/19/53/do-you-have-a-hormonal-imbalance

Down Dog | Great Yoga Anywhere. (n.d.). Down Dog | Great Yoga Anywhere. https://downdogapp.com/

Embracing Nutrition. (2019, September 10). Happiness begins in the gut. Embracing Nutrition & Functional Medicine. https://embracingnutrition.co.uk/happiness-begins-in-the-gut/

Enos, E. (2016, May 8). *Spring Detox: The Power of Parsley & Cilantro.* Denver Naturopathic Clinic | Healing Roots. https://healingrootsclinic.com/spring-detox-parsley-cilantro/

Environmental Working Group. (2019). *Dirty Dozen[TM] Fruits and Vegetables with the Most Pesticides.* Ewg.org. https://ewg.org/foodnews/dirty-dozen.php

Eske, J. (2019, April 9). *Is mineral water more healthful? Benefits and side effects.* medicalnewstoday.com. https://medicalnewstoday.com/articles/324910

ExRx.net : Exercise & Health Quotes. (n.d.). Exrx.net. Retrieved August 31, 2022, from https://exrx.net/ExInfo/Quotes

Falconer, A. (2020, March 5). *Gut Health Cleanse: Should You Detox Your Gut?* Healthpath. https://healthpath.com/gut-health/gut-health-cleanse-detox-your-gut/

5 Exercises That Aid in Optimal Digestive Health. (2022, May 18). Allied Digestive Health. https://allieddigestivehealth.com/5-exercises-that-aid-in-optimal-digestive-health/

Francis, G. (2021, March 3). *Want to Be Healthier? Start by Cleaning up Your Liver and Gut.* Veracityselfcare.com. https://veracityselfcare.com/en/knowledge/body/gut-liver-health

Gardiner, A. (2021, July 15). *Poor gut health can lead to these chronic diseases.* MDLinx. https://mdlinx.com/article/poor-gut-health-can-lead-to-these-chronic-diseases/1TzMRXobWPsfZfqAKgoVMM

Giambò, F., Teodoro, M., Costa, C., & Fenga, C. (2021). *Toxicology and Microbiota: How Do Pesticides Influence Gut Microbiota? A Review.* International Journal of Environmental Research and Public Health, 18(11), 5510. https://doi.org/10.3390/ijerph18115510

Gunnars, K. (2019, December 12). *Are Vegetable and Seed Oils Bad for Your Health?* Healthline. https://healthline.com/nutrition/are-vegetable-and-seed-oils-bad#what-they-are

Gut Cleanse: How to Cleanse the Gut to Improve Gut Health? (2020, May 5). phwcbermuda.com. https://phwcbermuda.com/best-gut-cleanse#:~:text=A%20gut%20cleansing%2C%20also%20known

Gut Health Cheat Sheet – The Healthy Life Foundation. (2020, December). The Healthy Life Foundation. https://thehealthylifefoundation.org/gut-health-cheat-sheet/

Gut Microbiome Testing for Weight Loss & Health. (2019). Viome. https://viome.com/

Hanka, S. (2022, January 3). *25 Gut Health Foods You Should Eat More Of.* trifectanutrition.com. https://trifectanutrition.com/blog/25-gut-health-foods-you-should-eat-more-of

Hanna, C. (2021, June 29). *Thirteen Ways To Improve Gut Health: Research-Backed Tips.* Healthpath. https://healthpath.com/gut-health/improve-gut-health/#:~:text=One%20of%20the%20best%20ways%20to%20improve%20your

Harvard Health Publishing. (2019). *The gut-brain connection - Harvard Health.* Harvard Health; Harvard Health. https://health.harvard.edu/diseases-and-conditions/the-gut-brain-connection

Health Benefits of Eating Raw Sprouts. (2021, March 3). Cleveland Clinic. https://health.clevelandclinic.org/what-are-the-health-benefits-and-risks-of-eating-sprouts/#:~:text=The%20types%20of%20sprouts&text=Bean%20and%20pea%20sprouts%3A%20These

Hills, J. (2019, April 3). *5 Worst Inflammatory Foods to Avoid If You Have Joint Pain According to Science.* Healthy and Natural World. https://healthyandnaturalworld.com/inflammatory-foods/

Hopes, S. (2022, July 18). *Yoga for digestion: How it works.* Livescience.com. https://livescience.com/yoga-for-digestion

https://cancer.gov/publications/dictionaries/cancer-terms/def/immune-function. (2011, February 2). cancer.gov. https://cancer.gov/publications/dictionaries/cancer-terms/def/immune-function

Ilchi Lee Quotes. (n.d.). BukRate. Retrieved August 29, 2022, from https://bukrate.com/quote/1703768

Is It Better to Drink Cold Water or Room Temperature Water? (n.d.). MedicineNet. Retrieved August 27, 2022, from https://medicinenet.com/drink_cold_water_or_room_temperature_water/article.htm

Jackson, H. (2018, July 12). *How to Get Back in the Habit of Working Out | Fitness 19 Gyms.* Fitness 19. https://fitness19.com/how-to-get-back-in-the-habit-of-working-out/

Kassel, G. (2018, November 12). *How exercise affects cortisol—the stress hormone.* Well+Good. https://wellandgood.com/exercise-cortisol/

Kellman, R. (2022, June 2). *Best Supplements for Your Gut, Says Physician.* Eat This Not That. https://eatthis.com/news-best-supplements-for-your-gut-says-physician/

Kozmor, T. (n.d.). *3 Ways Exercise Affects the Gut.* Ixcela. Retrieved August 31, 2022, from https://ixcela.com/resources/3-ways-exercise-affects-the-gut.html#:~:text=Exercising%20keeps%20sickness%20at%20bay.&text=(1)%20These%20gut%20microbiota%2C

Kubala, J. (2021, August 9). *7 Proven Health Benefits of Rhodiola Rosea.* Healthline. https://healthline.com/nutrition/rhodiola-rosea#TOC_TITLE_HDR_10

La Forge, T. (2021, December 10). *Here's How You Can Use Herbs to Relieve Anxiety.* Healthline. https://healthline.com/health/mental-health/herbs-for-stress-recipe#what-they-are

Leaky Gut Syndrome. (2022, April 6). Cleveland Clinic. https://my.clevelandclinic.org/health/diseases/22724-leaky-gut-syndrome#:~:text=Leaky%20gut%20syndrome%20is%20a%20theory%20that%20intestinal%20permeability%20is

Lemon balm Information | Mount Sinai - New York. (n.d.). Mount Sinai Health System. https://mountsinai.org/health-library/herb/lemon-balm#:~:text=Lemon%20balm%20(Melissa%20officinalis)%2C

Lewis, S. (2020, September 9). *Probiotics and Prebiotics: What's the Difference?* Healthline. https://healthline.com/nutrition/probiotics-and-prebiotics#bottom-line

Lindemann, B. (2016, August 14). *Why Dairy Might be Causing Your Digestive Distress.* Bella Lindemann. https://bellalindemann.com/blog/dairy-digestive-distress

Link, R. (2017, October 18). *8 Fermented Foods to Boost Digestion and Health.* Healthline; Healthline Media. https://healthline.com/nutrition/8-fermented-foods

MasterHealth Staff. (2022, February 7). *Dr. Frank Lipman: How to Heal Your Gut & Restore Gut Health.* MasterHealth. https://masterhealth.care/articles/how-to-heal-your-gut-restore-gut-health/

McDonald, E. (2020, September 4). *What foods cause or reduce inflammation?* uchicagomedicine.org. https://uchicagomedicine.org/forefront/gastrointestin al-articles/what-foods-cause-or-reduce-inflammation

Mindset Can Directly Affect Your Digestive System. (2018, January 9). The Real Life RD. https://thereallife-rd.com/2018/01/mindset-digestive-health/

Mudge, L. (2022, March 29). *What is gut health and why is it important?* Livescience.com. https://livescience.com/what-is-gut-health-and-why-is-it-important#section-why-is-gut-health-important

Nichols, H. (2020, March 12). *Estrogen: Functions, uses, and imbalances.* medicalnewstoday.com. https://medicalnewstoday.com/articles/277177#:~:tex t=In%20females%2C%20it%20helps%20develop

Orenstein, B. W. (2015, July 27). *10 Best and Worst Oils for Your Health.* EverydayHealth.com. https://everydayhealth.com/news/best-worst-oils-health/

Parch, L. A. (2020, June). *Ashwagandha Benefits | Everyday Health.* EverydayHealth.com. https://everydayhealth.com/diet-nutrition/the-benefits-of-ashwagandha/

Patino, E. (2020, June 10). *Signs of an Unhealthy Gut and What You Can Do About It | Everyday Health.* EverydayHealth.com. https://everydayhealth.com/digestive-health/signs-of-unhealthy-gut-and-how-to-fix-it/

Popa, B. (2019, May 17). *Glutathione: The "Master" Antioxidant.* Core Med Science. https://coremedscience.com/blogs/wellness/glutathio ne-the-master-antioxidant

Raman, R. (2018, July 14). *14 Healthy Whole-Grain Foods (Including Gluten-Free Options).* Healthline. https://healthline.com/nutrition/whole-grain-foods#TOC_TITLE_HDR_10

Richards, L. (2020, April 3). *Herbs for anxiety: 9 calming options.* medicalnewstoday.com. https://medicalnewstoday.com/articles/herbs-for-anxiety#lavender

Rossi, M. (2020, November 22). *How to get your gut-loving 30 plant points a week.* The Gut Health Doctor. https://theguthealthdoctor.com/how-to-get-your-gut-loving-30-plant-points-a-week/

Roth, I. (2018, June 11). *Mayo Clinic Minute: Which is better for losing weight - diet or exercise?* Mayo Clinic News Network. https://newsnetwork.mayoclinic.org/discussion/mayo-clinic-minute-which-is-better-for-losing-weight-diet-or-exercise/#:~:text=%22For%20weight%20loss%2C%2 0diet%20seems

Ruscio, M. (2021, August 31). *Use an Elimination Diet to Heal Your Gut, Brain, and Skin.* Drruscio.com. https://drruscio.com/elimination-diet/

Saumya, J. (2022, May 29). *World Digestive Health Day 2022: Theme, History, Significance, Quotes, Foods to Improve Digestion and more.* Jagran TV. https://jagrantv.com/en-show/world-digestive-health-day-2022-theme-history-significance-quotes-foods-to-improve-digestion-and-more-rc1031681

Schetler, A. (2021, April 6). *The 80/20 Rule—Eat Healthy and Have Your Cake, Too!* virtua.org. https://virtua.org/articles/the-80-20-rule-eat-healthy-and-have-your-cake-too#:~:text=The%2080%2F20%20rule%20is%20a%20guide%20for%20your%20everyday

Scott, E. (2020, December 12). *The Benefits of Box Breathing for Stress Management.* Verywell Mind. https://verywellmind.com/the-benefits-and-steps-of-box-breathing 4159900#:~:text=Box%20breathing%2C%20also%20known%20as

Scott, E. (2021, July 29). *17 Highly Effective Stress Relievers.* Verywell Mind; Verywellmind. https://verywellmind.com/tips-to-reduce-stress-3145195

Scott, L. A. (n.d.). *Gut Health and Hormones.* Leigh Ann Scott MD, Las Colinas, Irving TX. https://leighannscottmd.com/additional-testing/gut-health-and-hormones/#:~:text=When%20gut%20health%20isn

Segre, J. (2022, August 18). *Microbiome.* Genome.gov. https://genome.gov/genetics-glossary/Microbiome

Self Care for Your Body and Mind - Three great ways to take care of yourself everyday. (2020, February 27). The RESTART® Program. https://therestartprogram.com/self-care-for-your-body-and-mind-three-great-ways-to-take-care-of-yourself-everyday/

Semeco, A. (2016, June 8). *The 19 Best Prebiotic Foods You Should Eat.* Healthline; Healthline Media. https://healthline.com/nutrition/19-best-prebiotic-foods

Signs of poor gut health. (n.d.). piedmont.org. https://piedmont.org/living-better/signs-of-poor-gut-health

Sohal, M. (n.d.). *allplants | Examples of whole foods | Whole foods health benefits.* Allplants.com. https://allplants.com/blog/lifestyle/why-choose-whole-foods

Spritzler, F. (2019, November 12). *6 Foods That Cause Inflammation.* Healthline. https://healthline.com/nutrition/6-foods-that-cause-inflammation#3.-Vegetable-and-seed-oils

Stuart, A. (2008, September 3). *Natural Colon Cleansing & Detox: Is It Necessary?* WebMD; WebMD. https://webmd.com/balance/guide/natural-colon-cleansing-is-it-necessary

Study shows how serotonin and a popular anti-depressant affect the gut's microbiota. (2019). ScienceDaily. https://sciencedaily.com/releases/2019/09/190906092809.htm

Talia. (2013, April 2). *Daily Bite [Say]: Take Care of Your Body via Jim Rohn.* Dash of Wellness. https://dashofwellness.com/daily-bite-say-take-care-your-body-via-jim-rohn/

That Good Gut. (n.d.). Ashleycarlsonco.teachable.com. Retrieved August 26, 2022, from https://ashleycarlsonco.teachable.com/p/that-good-gut

The Brain-Gut Connection. (2019). John Hopkins Medicine. https://hopkinsmedicine.org/health/wellness-and-prevention/the-brain-gut-connection

The Chalkboard Editorial Team. (2016, June 10). *9 Mindful Eating Tips For Better Digestion*. The Chalkboard. https://thechalkboardmag.com/9-mindful-eating-tips-better-digestion

The Seven Dimensions of Wellness for a Healthy and Happy Life. (2018, July 31). Jill Conyers. https://jillconyers.com/2018/07/dimensions-wellness-healthy-life/

The Truth About Dry Brushing. (2021, November 2). Cleveland Clinic. https://health.clevelandclinic.org/the-truth-about-dry-brushing-and-what-it-does-for-you/#:~:text=What%20is%20dry%20brushing%3F

Tinsley, G. (2018). *6 Benefits of Reishi Mushroom (Plus Side Effects and Dosage)*. Healthline. https://healthline.com/nutrition/reishi-mushroom-benefits

Valente, L. (2022, May 6). *7 Must-Eat Fermented Foods for a Healthy Gut*. EatingWell. https://eatingwell.com/article/281916/7-must-eat-fermented-foods-for-a-healthy-gut/

Vich Vila, A., Collij, V., Sanna, S., Sinha, T., Imhann, F., Bourgonje, A. R., Mujagic, Z., Jonkers, D. M. A. E., Masclee, A. A. M., Fu, J., Kurilshikov, A., Wijmenga, C., Zhernakova, A., & Weersma, R. K. (2020). *Impact of commonly used drugs on the composition and metabolic function of the gut microbiota*. Nature Communications, 11(1), 362. https://doi.org/10.1038/s41467-019-14177-z

Warner, J. (2009, November 13). *Dark Chocolate Takes Bite Out of Stress*. WebMD. https://webmd.com/balance/stress-management/news/20091113/dark-chocolate-takes-bite-out-of-

stress#:~:text=Researchers%20found%20that%20eatin
g%20the

Well + Good Editors. (2019, April 11). *Why women's gut health issues are often undiagnosed.* Well+Good. https://wellandgood.com/womens-gut-health-renew-life/

West, H. (2017, June 3). *20 Clever Tips to Eat Healthy When Eating Out.* Healthline. https://healthline.com/nutrition/20-healthy-tips-for-eating-out#TOC_TITLE_HDR_20

What to Know About Alternate-Nostril Breathing. (n.d.). WebMD. https://webmd.com/balance/what-to-know-about-alternate-nostril-breathing#:~:text=With%20this%20nostril%20covered%2C%20close

Yuka - Food & Cosmetic scanner. (n.d.). App Store. https://apps.apple.com/us/app/yuka-food-cosmetic-scanner/id1092799236